Nature's Healing Remedies

A Holistic Guide to Herbal Wellness & Vitality (Revised)

Herbal Wellness Series

Book One

Sage Meadows

Praise for Nature's Healing Remedies

Sage Meadows' tried-and-true, science-backed herbal book is a must-have for all holistic health enthusiasts! Each page is packed with highly transformative wisdom that will empower each reader to pave their way to increased vitality and an all-enveloping sense of well-being. This author's timeless insights acquired from their time in Yunnan, China, Africa, and beyond are evident. ***Nature's Healing Remedies*** serves as testament that the ancient ways and modern-day life can coexist harmoniously.

-Eva Xan, Best-Selling Poetry Book Editor & Author of *Esoterra*

This is a revised edition of the original work published in 2025. It includes updated content, formatting enhancements, and additional reflections.

www.avoypublishing.com

NOTE FROM THE AUTHOR

This Revised Edition represents a meaningful chapter in my personal journey—both as a writer and as someone committed to a life of peace, clarity, and emotional renewal. Since the original publication, I've revisited these pages with a fresh perspective and deeper calm, refining the message and honoring the insights shared by readers like you.

Whether you're discovering this book for the first time or returning for a second look, I hope these words offer you comfort, clarity, and a path toward ease.

With gratitude,

Sage Meadows

AVOY Publishing

AUTHOR'S OTHER WORKS

BY SAGE MEADOWS

- *Still Clear, Changes the Game. Your Story. Your Power. Your Clarity (Revised)*
- *Still Strong, Reclaiming Your Body, Your Energy, and Your Joy After 50 (Revised)*
- *Nature's Healing Remedies, A Holistic Guide to Herbal Wellness & Vitality (Color - Collector)*
- *Nature's Healing Remedies, Word Search*
- *Nature's Healing Remedies, Journal*

Visit other works by Sage Meadows at www.avoypublishing.com

Dedication

To the readers—may these words find you where you are and meet you where you need them most.

Acknowledgments

I am deeply grateful to my spouse, daughters, and son. Your unwavering love, support, and presence have been the constant light on this creative journey. Thank you for inspiring every verse and every moment of reflection.

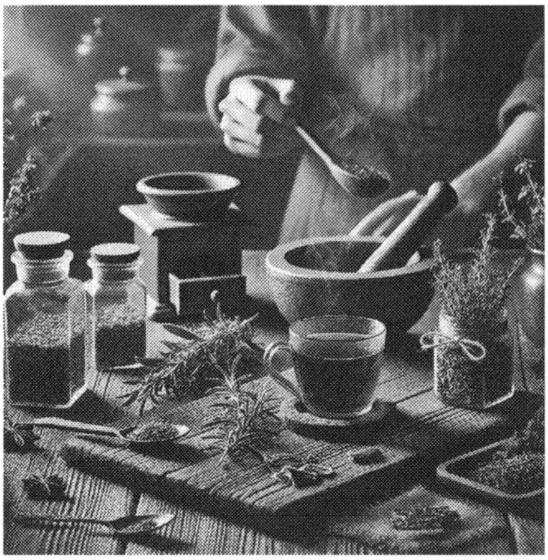

"Whether you're looking to alleviate chronic conditions, bolster your immune system, or adopt a more natural lifestyle, this book offers a reliable guide grounded in thorough research and practical insights."

Contents

Preface

As long as humans have walked the earth, we have turned to nature for healing. Long before modern medicine, our ancestors relied on plants to strengthen the body from within. Across every culture, from the rainforests to the mountain valleys, generations have passed down knowledge of nature's remedies, shaping a tradition of healing that remains as relevant today as it was centuries ago.

In our fast-paced, modern world, people often overlook this wisdom. Synthetic solutions frequently overshadow natural ones, quick fixes replace long-term wellness, and we have become disconnected from the source of healing surrounding us. But nature has never stopped offering its gifts. The question is—are we ready to listen again?

This book, ***Nature's Healing Remedies: A Holistic Guide to Herbal Wellness & Vitality***, invites us to rediscover what has always been there: the power of plants to support, nurture, and enhance our well-being. It is not about rejecting modern advancements but about restoring balance—integrating the time-tested benefits of herbal medicine into daily life in a way that is practical, effective, and accessible to all.

These pages teach you how to recognize, prepare, and use herbs in ways that honor their potency and tradition. Whether you are taking your first steps into the world of herbal healing or expanding your knowledge, this guide will empower you to work with nature's pharmacy confidently and responsibly.

True healing is not just about treating symptoms—it is about strengthening the body, supporting the mind, and fostering a way of living that aligns with the natural world's rhythms. Herbal medicine is not a trend but a practice of patience, care, and connection. Once you begin this journey, it may change more than just your health—it deepens your relationship with the world around you.

I invite you to explore, experiment, and embrace nature's wisdom. May this book serve as a guide, a companion, and a reminder that everything we need to heal has always been within reach—growing quietly in the world around us.

With gratitude and green blessings,

Sage Meadows🌿✨

Introduction

"Herbal remedies, where ancient wisdom and modern science converge to unlock the keys to longevity, vitality, and holistic well-being."

High in the mist-laden mountains of Yunnan, China, I found myself in a world where ancient wisdom and modern life existed in delicate harmony. Strolling through a small village adorned with terraced gardens, I approached an older woman whose presence radiated warmth and wisdom. She carried a basket filled with freshly harvested herbs in her weathered hands, their fragrance a rich blend of earth and vitality. As she gently placed a sprig of medicinal leaves in my palm, I felt the weight of centuries of knowledge pass between us—an unspoken invitation to explore the profound relationship between humanity and the healing power of plants. This moment ignited a journey that would forever change my understanding of health and wellness, and I invite you to join me on this journey.

As we navigate a fast-paced world increasingly dominated by synthetic medications and quick-fix solutions, many seek solace in nature's apothecary. According to recent studies, nearly 40% of adults in the U.S. integrate complementary and alternative medicine into their lifestyles, with herbal remedies among the most trusted choices. This shift represents more than a passing trend—a return to the roots of healing, a reconnection with the wisdom generations before us relied upon for vitality and well-being.

Nature's Healing Remedies: A Holistic Guide to Herbal Wellness & Vitality is more than a guidebook—it is an invitation to rediscover the gifts of nature and reclaim control over your health. This book bridges the timeless traditions of herbal medicine with modern scientific understanding, empowering you with practical knowledge and confidence. Whether new to herbalism or have been practicing for years, this book will help you incorporate plant-based remedies into your daily routine and witness their positive effects.

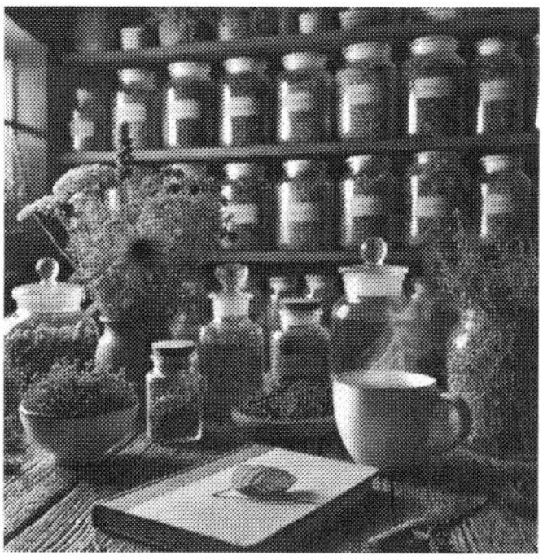

Throughout these pages, you will explore the intricate world of medicinal herbs, learning how to identify, source, and prepare them with precision and care. You will discover how to craft herbal teas that soothe and restore, salves that nourish the skin, and tinctures that harness the potent healing properties of plants. More than just recipes, this book delves into the scientific mechanisms that make herbal medicine effective, unlocking the secrets of plant compounds, their interactions with the body, and how they support natural healing processes.

My journey as an herbalist and wellness educator has taken me across the world—from the remote villages of China, where I immersed myself in the foundational concepts and practices that make up Traditional Chinese Medicine (TCM), to the rich herbal landscapes of Africa and Europe, and back to the untamed meadows of my homeland, where nature's pharmacy flourishes in abundance. With each experience, I have witnessed plant medicine's profound impact on human health, and I am honored to share this wisdom with you.

This is your guide to seeking relief from chronic ailments, striving to build a resilient immune system, or embracing a more natural way of life.

For many, stepping into the world of herbal medicine can feel overwhelming. The terminology may seem foreign, and the sheer volume of information—often conflicting—can be daunting. Words like phytochemicals, adaptogens, and bioavailability can deter even the most enthusiastic learner. That is why this book has been crafted with clarity and accessibility in mind, offering a structured, easy-to-follow guide for integrating herbal healing into your life. Whether you seek relief from chronic ailments, strive to build a resilient immune system, or wish to embrace a more natural way of living, this book will be your trusted companion, grounded in research and practical application.

As you turn these pages, I encourage you to approach herbal medicine with an open heart and curiosity. Trust in nature's intelligence and your body's innate ability to heal. Connecting more deeply with the plants that sustain us enhances our health and develops a profound appreciation for the natural world.

Now, let us step into the timeless realm of herbal remedies, where ancient wisdom and modern science converge to unlock the keys to longevity, vitality, and holistic well-being. The path to natural healing begins here, and I am honored to walk along this path with you.

Foundations of Herbal Medicine

"Cornerstone of wellness"

Plants have been humanity's most trusted healing ally for thousands of years. Across every continent and civilization, herbal medicine has been a cornerstone of wellness, offering natural solutions to ailments and enhancing vitality. As we embark on this journey through the foundations of herbal medicine, we uncover the wisdom of the past, the science of the present, and the boundless potential for the future.

The Ancient Roots of Herbal Medicine

Before modern pharmaceuticals, our ancestors turned to nature's bounty for healing. The knowledge of medicinal plants was transmitted through generations and was often carefully preserved within families, monasteries, and indigenous communities. For example, ancient texts like the Egyptian Ebers Papyrus, composed over 3,500 years ago, describe remedies that utilized aloe vera, frankincense, and myrrh.

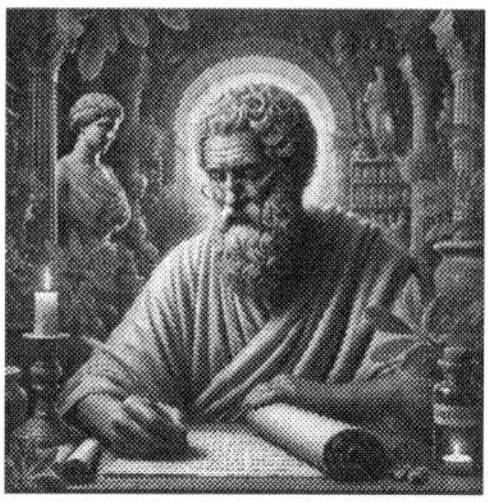

Greek physician Hippocrates

From the Greek physician Hippocrates, who emphasized the healing power of food and medicine, to medieval herbalists who preserved and safeguarded ancient wisdom, plant-based medicine has always been integral to human survival and progress. Deeply rooted in history, Traditional Chinese Medicine and Ayurveda have built sophisticated systems based on plant synergy, balance, and energetic healing. While many of these ancient remedies remain validated by modern science, they remind us of the innate connection between nature and well-being.

The Science Behind Herbal Medicine

Herbs are more than folklore; they are biologically active powerhouses with measurable effects on the Body.

Modern research has identified the phytochemicals—the active compounds responsible for a plant's medicinal properties. For example:

1. **Flavonoids** in herbs like chamomile and ginkgo biloba possess potent anti-inflammatory and antioxidant properties.
2. **Alkaloids** in plants such as goldenseal and echinacea contribute to immune support and antimicrobial benefits.
3. **Terpenes** are found in herbs like peppermint and rosemary. These compounds offer therapeutic effects, from mental clarity to digestive support.

Science continues to validate the use of herbs for various conditions, from heart health (hawthorn) to stress relief (ashwagandha) and digestive wellness (ginger). With increased global research, herbal medicine bridges the gap between tradition and modern science.

How Herbal Medicine Works in the Body

Unlike synthetic drugs, which often target one specific symptom or function, herbs work holistically with the Body's systems. They support balance rather than merely suppressing symptoms. Adaptogens, for instance, help the Body resist stress and restore equilibrium, while tonics nourish and strengthen bodily functions over time.

The Body absorbs herbs through various pathways:

1. **Digestive System** – absorbs medicinal compounds from teas, capsules, and tinctures.
2. **Respiratory System**—Aromatherapy (and herbal steams) deliver plant essences through inhalation, benefiting the lungs and nervous System.
3. **Topical Absorption** – Herbal salves, poultices, and oils penetrate the skin, aiding localized healing.

Understanding how herbs interact with the Body allows for more effective and personalized usage, making herbal medicine an adaptable tool for long-term wellness.

COMMON CONCERNS AND SAFETY IN HERBAL MEDICINE

As with healing, safety and proper use are essential. While herbs are generally gentler than pharmaceuticals, we must still use them with awareness. Considerations include:

1. **Herb-Drug Interactions** – Some herbs, like St. John's Wort, can alter the effectiveness of prescription medications.
2. **Dosage and Preparation** – The form in which an herb is used (tea, tincture, capsule) affects its potency and effectiveness.
3. **Sourcing and Purity** – Choosing organic, sustainably harvested herbs ensures maximum benefits and minimizes exposure to pesticides and contaminants.

Consulting qualified herbalists or integrative health practitioners can help tailor herbal use to individual needs, ensuring both efficacy and safety.

The Future of Herbal Healing

In today's fast-paced world, the wisdom of herbal medicine is experiencing a resurgence, further cementing its place in modern healthcare. As we explore this book further, we will explore how to seamlessly integrate herbs into our everyday routines, master preparation techniques, and discover the profound impact of herbal remedies on both Body and mind. The journey into herbal medicine is not just about knowledge—it's about reconnecting with nature and rediscovering the healing power within.

Understanding the Healing Potential of Herbs

With a strong foundation in herbal medicine laid, it's time to step into the heart of nature's healing wisdom. Now that we understand herbs' history, science, and role in holistic well-being, we must ask: *Which plants hold the most significant healing potential?* In the next chapter, we will explore some of the most potent medicinal herbs—learning to identify them, understand their properties, and harness their benefits for everyday health. Let's embark on this journey into the plant kingdom and unlock the secrets of nature's pharmacy.🌿✨

Where Ancient Wisdom and Modern Science Converge

"An empowering journey"

The Essence of Herbal Wisdom

Herbal medicine has woven itself into the fabric of human history, serving as a foundation of health and healing across cultures. People have turned to nature's apothecary from ancient to modern times to maintain wellness and combat ailments. To fully benefit from herbal remedies, it's essential to understand how to identify, cultivate, and use these resilient plants. This chapter delves into recognizing, identifying, and using herbal remedies properly to avoid adverse effects and embrace their wisdom.

The Art of Identifying Medicinal Herbs

The first step in integrating herbal remedies into daily life is the ability to recognize beneficial plants. Many medicinal herbs are hidden in plain sight—growing along pathways, fields, and backyards. However, the key to safe herbal use lies in proper identification.

Key Features to Observe:

1. **Leaf Shape and Texture:** Different herbs have unique leaf structures. For example, peppermint has deeply veined, serrated leaves that emit a cooling scent when crushed, while sage features soft, grey-green leaves with a robust, earthy aroma.
2. **Flower Characteristics:** A plant's flowers' color, shape, and size offer significant clues. Chamomile, for instance, bears daisy-like white petals with a yellow center, while echinacea displays a striking purple or pink cone surrounded by spiky petals.
3. **Aroma and Taste:** Many medicinal plants are distinguished by scent and flavor. Lavender exudes a sweet, floral fragrance, and rosemary releases a pine-like aroma when rubbed between the fingers.
4. **Growth Environment:** Certain plants thrive in specific conditions. Mullein, known for its respiratory benefits, prefers dry, sandy soils, whereas marshmallow root flourishes in wet, marshy areas.

Equipped with knowledge of these identifying features, herbalists can confidently distinguish medicinal herbs from lookalikes that may lack healing properties—or worse, be toxic.

Traditional Herbal Classifications and Their Significance

Ancient cultures categorized herbs based on their medicinal properties and energetic effects on the body. These classifications remain invaluable for modern herbalists:

1. **Adaptogens,** such as ashwagandha and ginseng, support the body's ability to handle stress and restore balance.
2. **Astringents:** blackberry leaves and witch hazel tighten tissues and reduce excessive secretions.

3. **Bitters:** dandelion and gentian stimulate digestion and enhance liver function.
4. **Demulcents:** slippery elm and marshmallow root soothe mucous membranes and reduce irritation.
5. **Diaphoretics:** elderflower and ginger promote sweating and aid detoxification.
6. **Nervines:** valerian and passionflower calm the Nervous system and improve relaxation.

VISUAL GUIDE TO KEY MEDICINAL HERBS

Understanding and identifying medicinal herbs is crucial for their practical use. While this book provides valuable insights into 25 essential herbs, including their therapeutic applications and growing environments, we encourage readers to visit our website for a detailed visual guide. You'll find images and additional information to help you confidently recognize and utilize these herbal allies in your daily wellness practices.

IDENTIFYING 25 KEY HERBS

Across the world, herbalists have come to rely on specific plants for their consistent healing properties. Passed down through generations, these time-tested botanicals have earned their place in traditional and modern medicine. Below are 25 herbs that are both effective and relatively easy to identify in their natural habitats or gardens.

Chamomile – Known for its calming effects, it is easy to recognize chamomile's daisy-like flowers with white petals and a yellow center. It thrives in sunny fields, and its apple-like scent distinguishes it from similar plants.

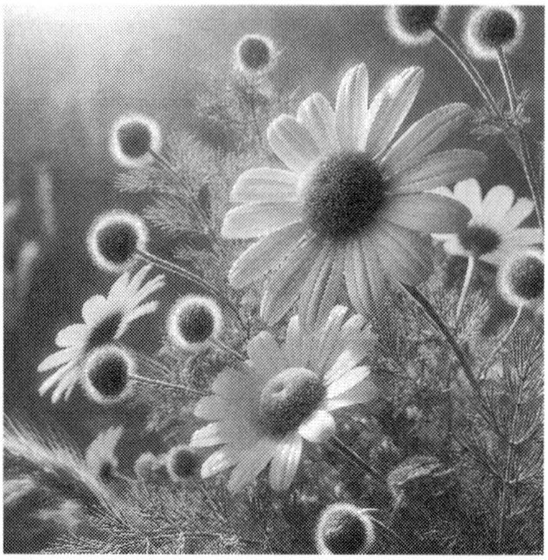

A blooming chamomile plant in a sunlit field showcases its delicate white petals, bright yellow center, and feathery green leaves.

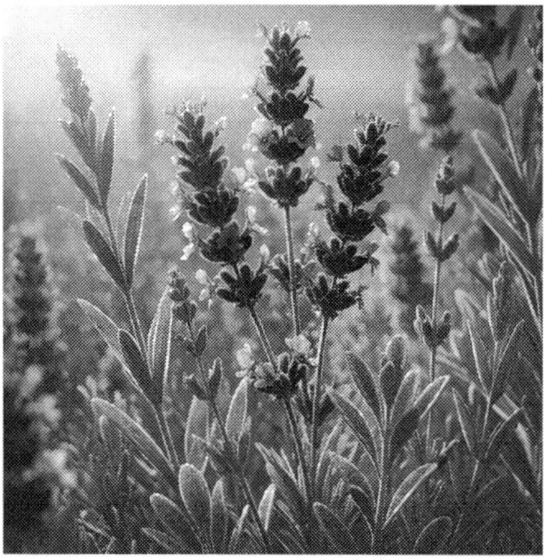

Lavender *– With its vibrant purple flowers and sweet fragrance, lavender is a staple for relaxation and skincare. It flourishes in dry conditions and is easily identified by its slender, grey-green leaves.*

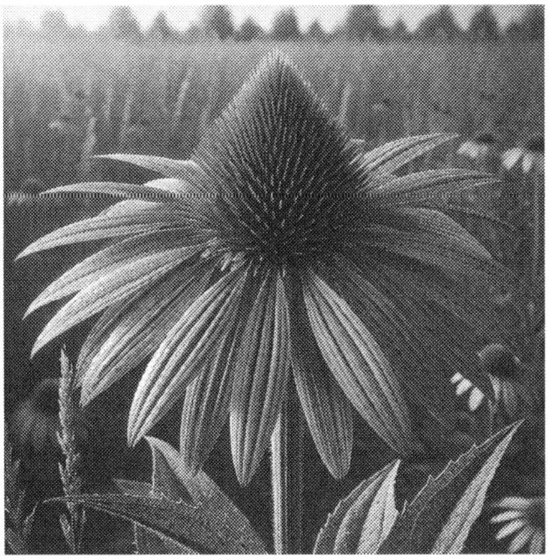

***Echinacea** (Coneflower) – A striking herb with pink or purple petals surrounding a spiky cone, echinacea is renowned for its immune-boosting properties. It grows in prairies and gardens, standing tall with rigid, coarse leaves.*

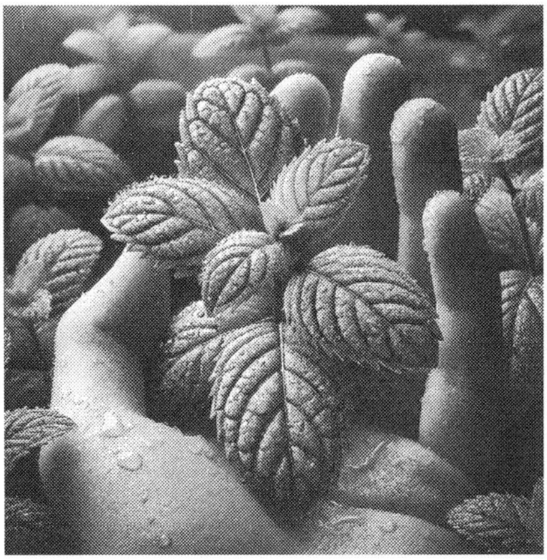

Peppermint—The deeply veined, serrated peppermint leaves release a cool, refreshing scent when crushed. This plant spreads quickly and is often found in damp areas.

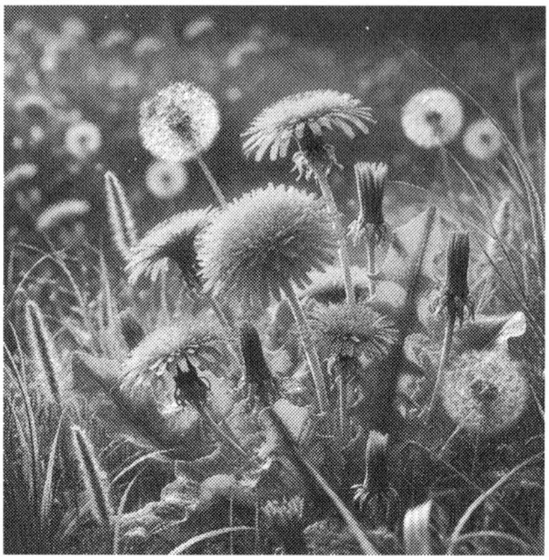

Dandelion – With bright yellow flowers and deeply toothed leaves, dandelions are more than weeds—they are liver-supporting powerhouses.

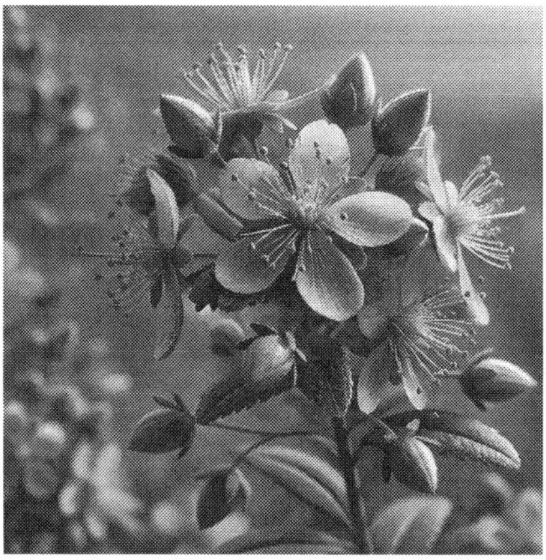

St. John's Wort – Recognizable by its small yellow flowers, this plant is widely used for mood support. When the flowers are crushed, they release a red-colored oil.

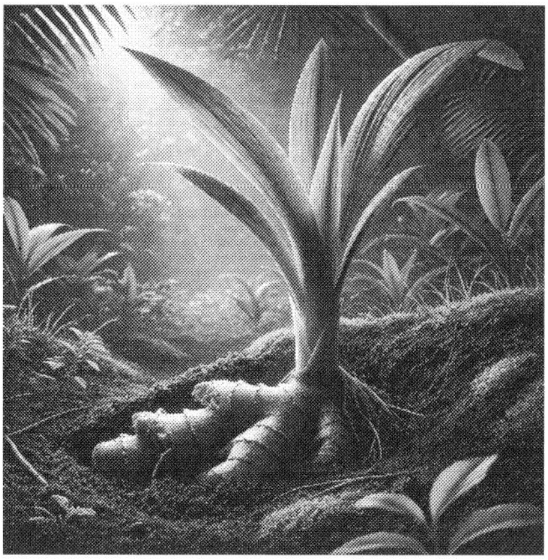

Ginger – The root of this plant is the most valuable part. Ginger is distinguished by its grass-like leaves and aromatic rhizomes found underground.

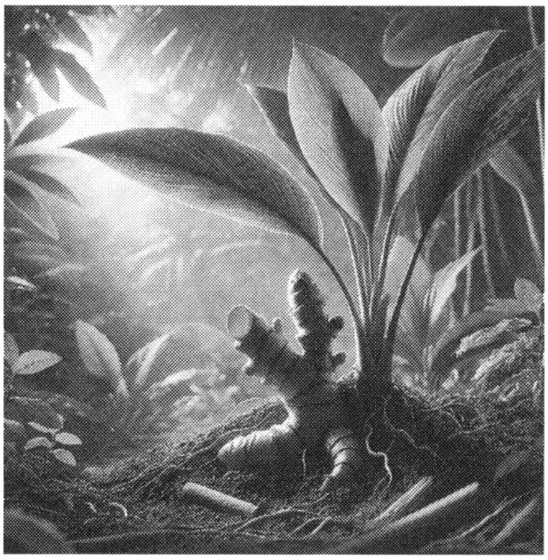

Turmeric – Often confused with ginger, turmeric's deep orange rhizome is packed with anti-inflammatory compounds. It thrives in warm, humid climates.

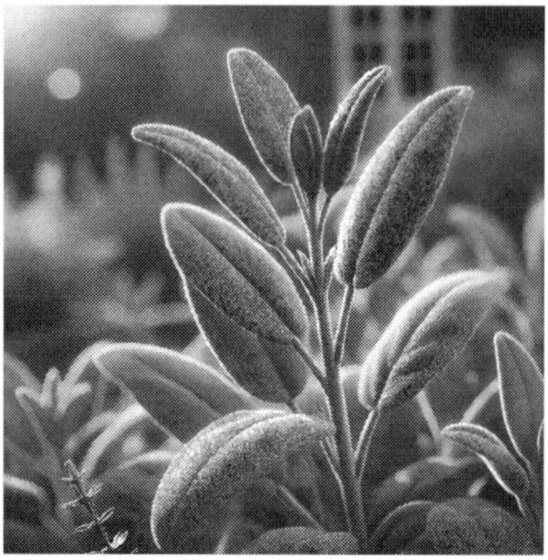

Sage—This herb features soft, grey-green leaves and a robust, earthy aroma. It has long been used in cooking and medicine.

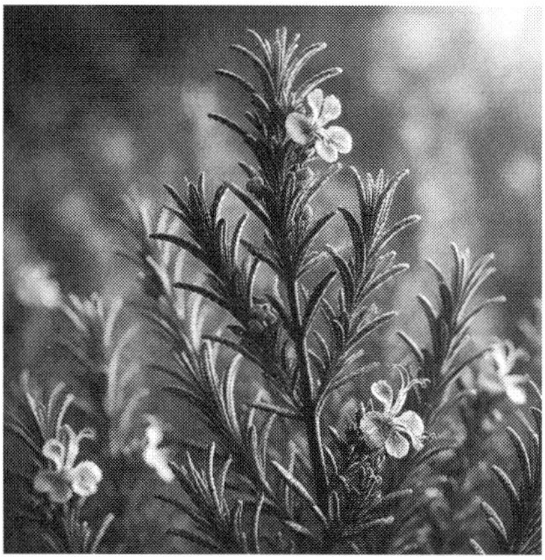

Rosemary – With needle-like leaves and a piney scent, rosemary is a potent antioxidant and memory-enhancing herb.

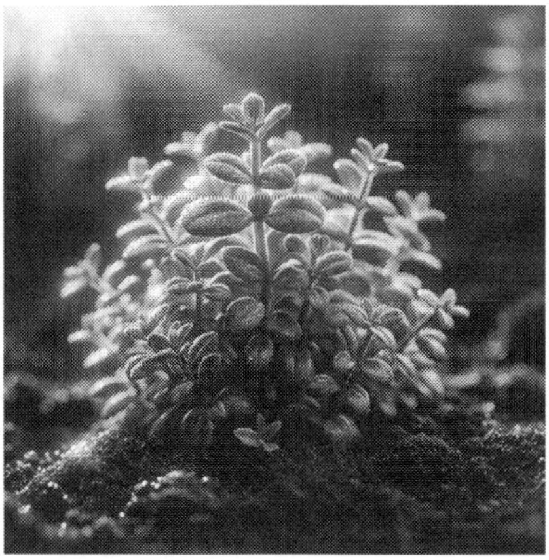

Thyme – A small, woody herb with tiny aromatic leaves, thyme is often used for respiratory health and culinary purposes.

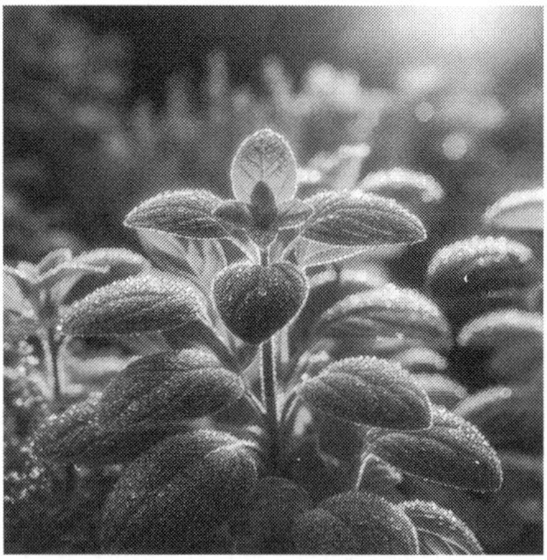

Oregano – Recognized by its robust flavor and small oval leaves, oregano is a powerful antimicrobial herb.

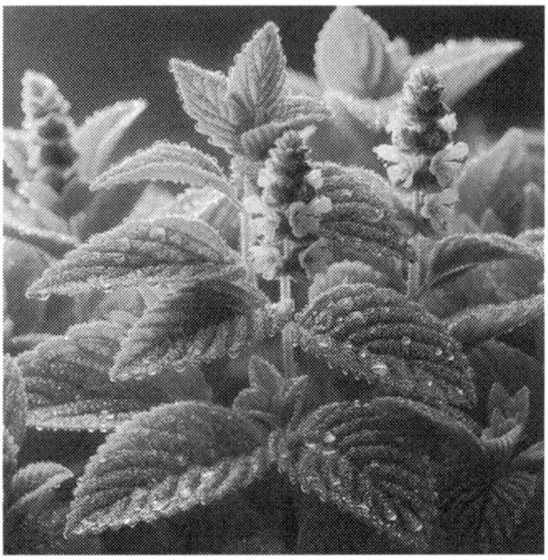

Lemon Balm – A member of the mint family, lemon balm has heart-shaped leaves and a bright citrus scent, making it a favorite for stress relief and digestion.

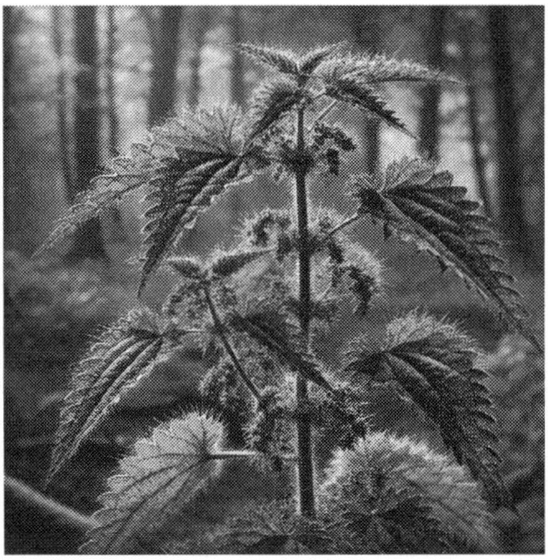

Nettle – Identified by its serrated leaves and fine stinging hairs, nettle is rich in nutrients and supports immune and urinary health.

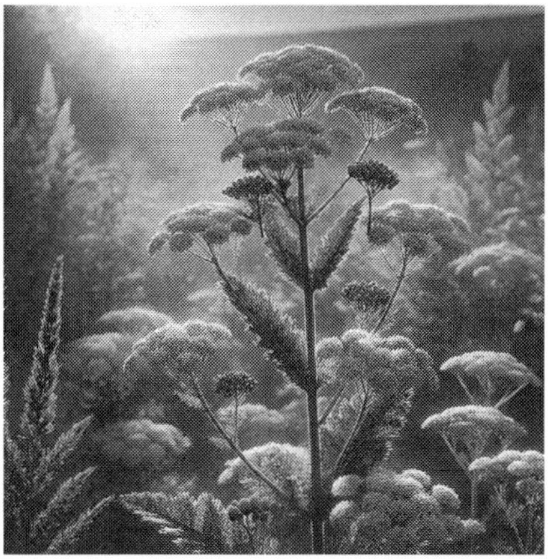

Yarrow – A medicinal plant with feathery leaves and clusters of tiny white or pink flowers, yarrow is used for wound healing and circulation support.

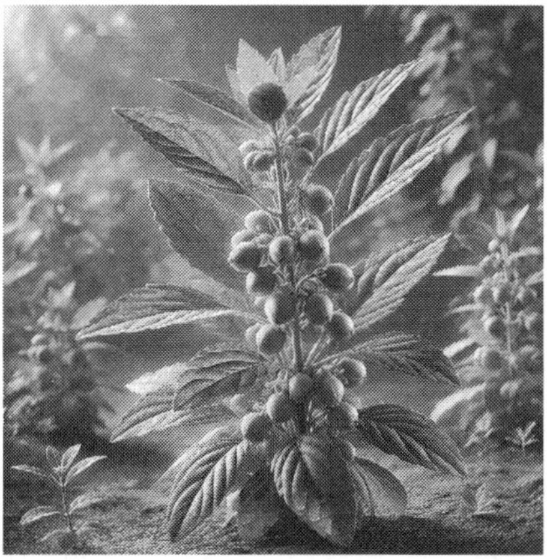

Ashwagandha—This adaptogenic herb with small green leaves and red berries is prized for its stress-reducing and rejuvenating properties.

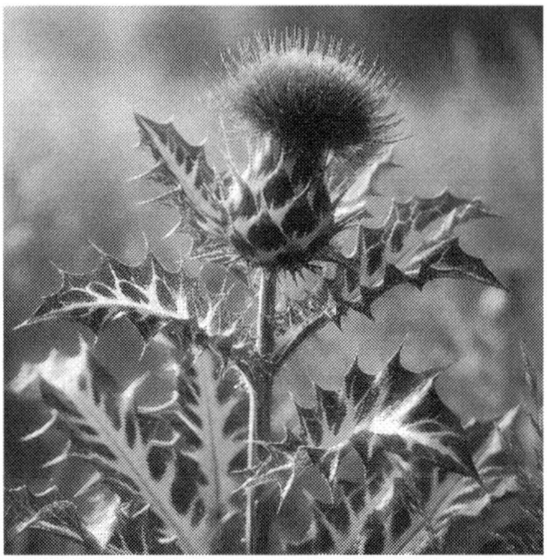

Milk Thistle – Recognized by its purple flowers and spiky leaves, milk thistle is widely used to support liver health.

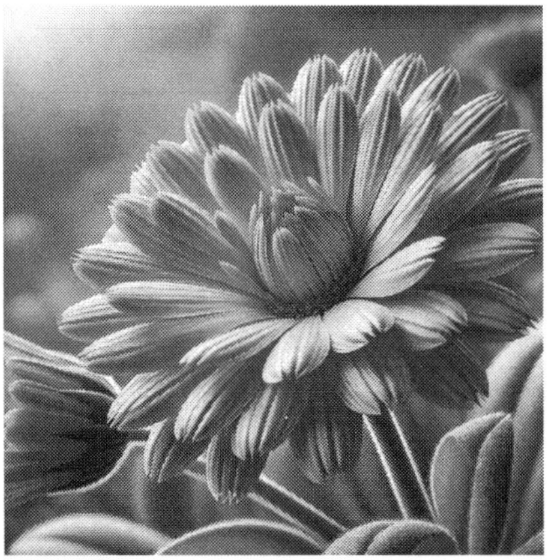

Calendula – A bright orange or yellow flower known for its skin-soothing and anti-inflammatory properties.

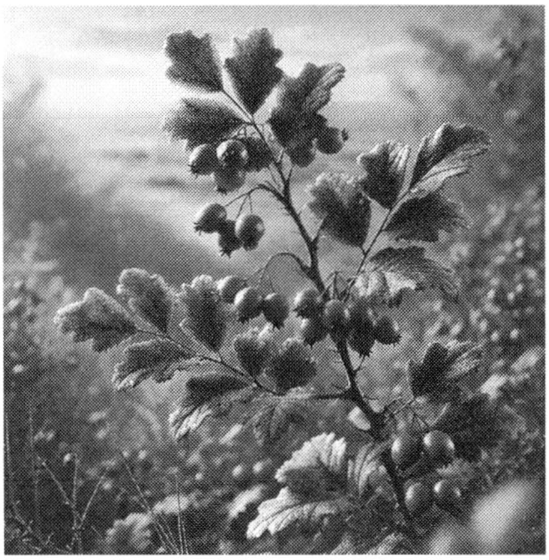

Hawthorn – A tree with clusters of small red berries, hawthorn is used for heart health and blood circulation.

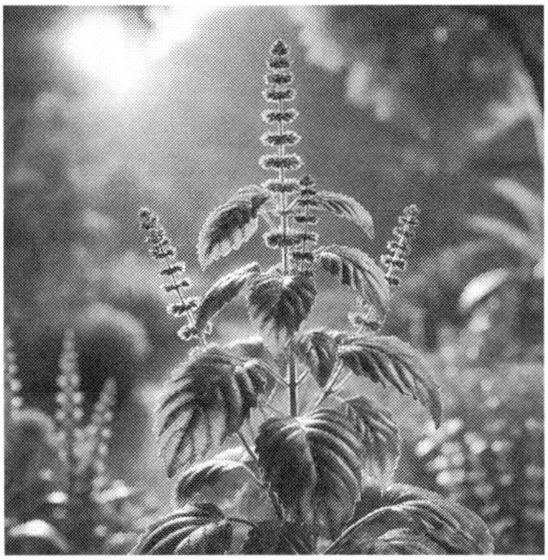

Holy Basil (Tulsi) – A revered plant in Ayurveda, tulsi has slightly serrated leaves and a spicy clove-like aroma, often used for stress relief.

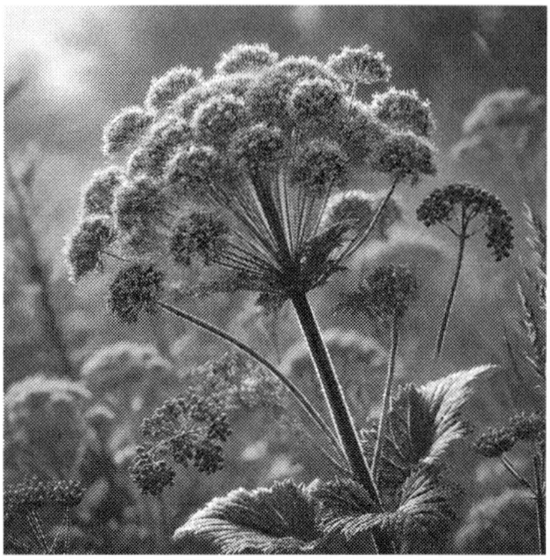

Valerian – A plant with clusters of small pink or white flowers, valerian root is well known for its calming and sleep-inducing properties.

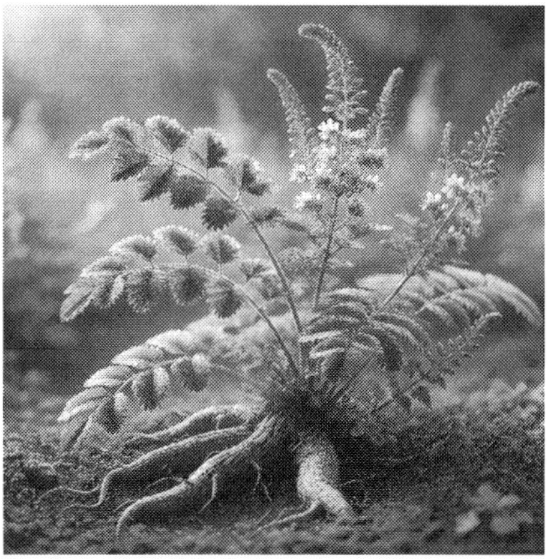

Licorice Root – A sweet-tasting root with anti-inflammatory and adrenal-supportive benefits.

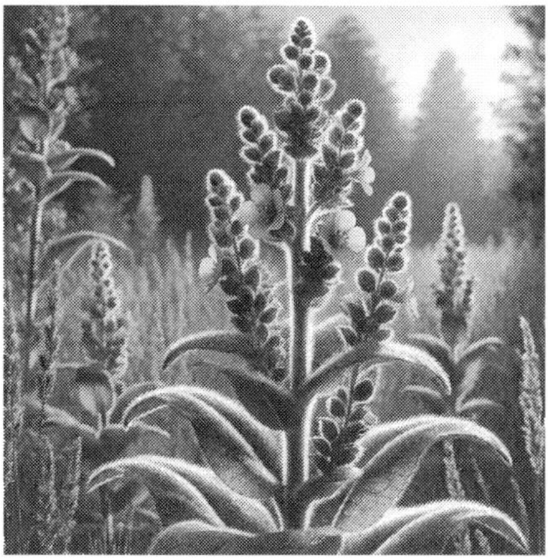

Mullein – A tall plant with soft, fuzzy leaves, mullein is commonly used for lung and respiratory support.

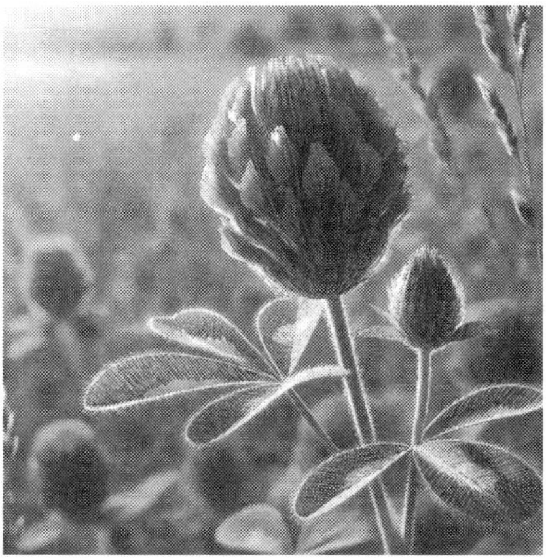

Red Clover – Recognizable by its rounded pinkish-purple flower heads, red clover is used for hormone balance and detoxification.

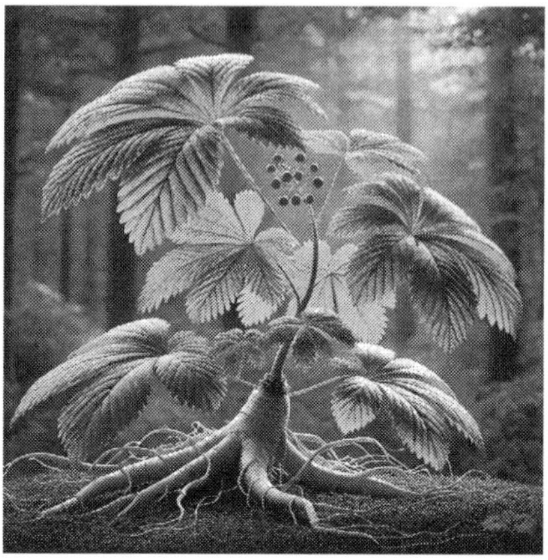

Ginseng – A root with a distinct forked shape, ginseng is an adaptogen that enhances energy and mental clarity.

Safety in Herbal Medicine: Essential Guidelines

While herbs offer powerful therapeutic benefits, we must use them with care and responsibility. Proper education on herbal safety prevents potential side effects and ensures optimal results.

Key Safety Considerations:

1. **Accurate Identification:** Mistaking one plant for another can lead to adverse effects. Always verify an herb's identity through multiple sources.
2. **Dosage Awareness:** Like pharmaceutical medicines, herbs have recommended dosages. Consuming too much can result in toxicity or unintended interactions.
3. **Understanding Contraindications:** Certain herbs are unsuitable for individuals with specific health conditions. For instance, licorice root should be avoided by those with high blood pressure.
4. **Interactions with Medications:** Some herbs affect how medications work in the body. St. John's Wort, commonly used for mood support, can have unintended consequences,

such as reduced contraceptive protection or altered mental health management.

5. **Quality Matters:** Organic, high-quality herbs ensure purity and potency, free from contaminants like pesticides or heavy metals

By adhering to these safety principles, individuals can confidently incorporate herbal remedies into their wellness routines.

Sourcing and Growing Your Medicinal Herbs

Growing medicinal herbs provides self-sufficiency and quality assurance for those seeking a deeper connection with their remedies. Many healing plants are easy to cultivate at home with minimal effort.

Best Herbs for Home Cultivation:

1. **Chamomile:** Grows well in small garden plots or containers; prized for its calming effects.
2. **Lavender:** Thrives in well-drained soil and sunlight; excellent for relaxation and skincare.
3. **Peppermint:** Spreads quickly and flourishes damply, aiding digestion.
4. **Echinacea:** Hardy and resilient, offering immune-boosting benefits.
5. **Lemon Balm:** Ideal for soothing nerves and enhancing mood.

Cultivating these herbs fosters a sustainable approach to herbal medicine while ensuring a readily available supply of potent plant allies.

Harvesting and Preserving Herbs for Maximum Potency

To maintain the highest medicinal quality, we should harvest them at the right time and appropriately preserve them.

1. **Best Time to Harvest:** We should pick the flowers when they are in full bloom, the leaves when they are vibrant and green, and the roots in late autumn when their nutrient content peaks.
2. **Drying Methods:** Air-drying in a shaded area preserves essential oils, while dehydrators speed up the process without compromising potency.
3. **Storage Techniques:** Herbs should be stored in airtight glass containers away from light and heat to retain their medicinal properties.

Proper harvesting and storage techniques extend the shelf life of herbs, ensuring their effectiveness for months or even years.

Embracing the Herbal Path

Identifying, growing, and safely using medicinal plants is an empowering journey that reconnects individuals with nature's healing gifts. By incorporating herbal wisdom into daily life, we honor the ancient traditions that have sustained human health for generations. Whether through a simple cup of chamomile tea, a soothing lavender salve, or a carefully cultivated home garden, the power of plants is ever-present, waiting to be nurtured and restored. In the next chapter, we will look at specific herb profiles and their diverse applications, guiding us further along the path of natural healing.🌿✨

The Art and Science of Herbal Preparation

"Mastering herbal preparations is both a science and an art."

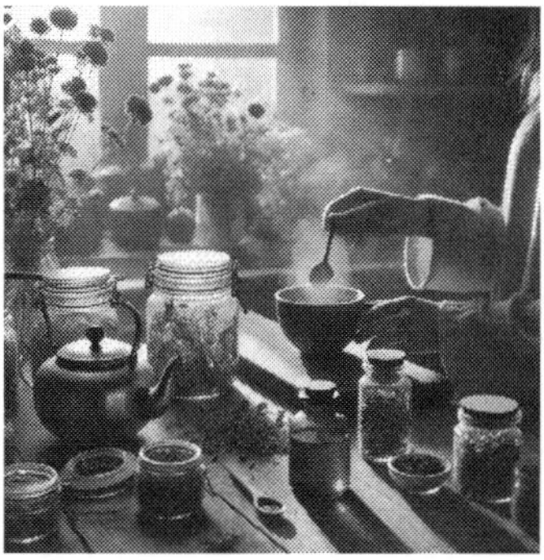

I watched a friend prepare a soothing herbal tea with practiced grace in a sunlit kitchen with rich, fresh, and dried herb aromas. The wooden countertops bore vibrant rosemary sprigs, delicate chamomile blossoms, and aromatic mint leaves while a gently steaming kettle filled the air with warmth. Each movement was deliberate as she measured, crushed, and blended the herbs, crafting a remedy steeped in generations of wisdom. She recalled how her grandmother would brew similar infusions, using the time-honored knowledge of plant medicine to heal and nourish the body. This simple act of herbal preparation, an ancient yet accessible art, serves as a direct link to nature's profound healing potential, grounding us in the harmony of the natural world.

A friend carefully measures loose herbs into a teacup while a steaming teapot sits nearby. Glass jars filled with botanical ingredients line the table, enhancing the traditional and calming atmosphere.

Crafting Herbal Teas: Infusions and Decoctions Explained

Herbal infusions and decoctions are cornerstone practices in herbal medicine, each tailored to harness the unique medicinal qualities of varying plant materials. Infusions, often celebrated for their gentle extraction process, are ideally suited for the more fragile parts of plants, such as leaves, flowers, and delicate stems. This method meticulously draws out the essential oils and therapeutic compounds without degrading their potency, making it perfect for plants whose virtues lie in their aromatic and volatile constituents. Decoctions extract the strong, resilient qualities of more demanding plant parts like roots, bark, and seeds. Decoctions break down these hardy materials through a prolonged simmering, releasing their dense healing properties into the water.

This method is particularly effective for extracting deep-seated, potent compounds that are not easily accessible through simple infusion. "By following this step, you fully realize the medicinal strength of the more rigid plant parts. Both techniques, infusions, and decoctions, are fundamental to extracting the vast array of medicinal properties plants offer. They provide a versatile framework for creating potent herbal remedies that address various therapeutic effects, from soothing and aromatic to profoundly restorative and healing.

Infusions: The Gentle Art of Herbal Tea

Infusions, a hallmark of herbal preparation, are particularly effective for processing the more delicate aspects of plants, including their leaves, flowers, and delicate stems. This method, also known as steeping, delicately coaxes out the beneficial properties of these plant parts through immersion in hot water. Unlike the vigorous extraction methods required for more complex materials, gently steeping persuades the release of essential oils and therapeutic agents without diminishing their potency. This process mirrors the making of traditional tea, where the herb's essence is infused into the water, capturing its full aromatic and healing potential. The secret to a successful infusion lies in balancing temperature and time. The water should be hot enough to facilitate extraction yet not so hot that it degrades the delicate compounds within the herbs.

This subtle art of infusion preserves the integrity and full spectrum of benefits offered by the more tender parts of the plant, making it an essential technique for any herbalist. The infusion process is simple:

1. Select High-Quality Herbs – Choose fresh or dried herbs known for their therapeutic benefits.
2. Heat the Water – Bring water to a gentle boil (around 200°F or 93°C).
3. Steep the Herbs: Pour hot water over the herbs and let them steep for 5 to 15 minutes, adjusting the time for your desired strength.
4. Cover to Retain Aromatics – Placing a lid over the infusion helps preserve essential oils.
5. After steeping or cooking the herbs in water to extract their beneficial properties, you should filter out the plant material using a sieve or cheesecloth or muslin cloth. The result is a clear liquid you can drink or use as intended, ensuring no unwanted bits of herbs are left behind.

Common herbs used in infusions include chamomile (calming), peppermint (digestive aid), and lemon balm (mood enhancer). The gentle extraction process makes infusions ideal for everyday consumption.

Decoctions: Extracting the Strength of Roots and Barks

Decoctions are an ancient practice meticulously designed to unlock the potent medicinal qualities of the plant kingdom's more resilient members—roots, bark, and hard seeds. This method goes beyond mere steeping, requiring a more intense process of simmering these more challenging plant materials. This process thoroughly extracts the dense, healing compounds deeply embedded within the herbs. A decoction is particularly adept at breaking down the cell walls of these hardy substances, thereby releasing their full spectrum of therapeutic properties into the water. This technique is essential for accessing herbal medicine's robust, often grounding elements that are not readily available through lighter extraction methods, such as infusions. Through the careful application of heat and time, decoctions make available the earth's deep-seated restorative powers, offering a powerful medium for the body's healing and nourishment. This method requires sustained heat to produce a decoction; take the following steps:

1. Measure the Herbs – Use approximately one tablespoon of dried roots or bark per cup of water.
2. Simmer Gently—Place herbs in a pot, submerge in water, slowly heat to a gentle boil, then reduce to a simmer.
3. Cook for 20-60 Minutes – The duration depends on the toughness of the plant material.
4. Strain and Store –Cool before straining into a jar for storage.

Popular decoction herbs include ginger (digestive aid), cinnamon (circulatory support), and echinacea (immune booster). Decoctions are especially effective for drawing out plant tannins, alkaloids, and minerals.

Tinctures: Concentrated Herbal Extracts

Tinctures are one of the most potent and enduring herbal extracts, meticulously preserved through alcohol, glycerin, or vinegar. This method of preservation not only extends the shelf life of the herbal properties but enhances the extract's concentration, making tinctures a potent tool in the herbalist's arsenal. They offer a practical and efficient means to integrate the profound benefits of herbal medicine into daily health routines. With just a few drops, these concentrated extracts deliver the essence of herbs in a form that is easy to administer and adjust according to individual needs, proving an indispensable asset for those seeking to embrace the full spectrum of nature's healing capabilities. The basic steps for developing an alcohol-based or non-alcohol-based tincture are:

Alcohol-Based Tinctures

1. Choose the Herb – Select dried or fresh plant material suitable for extraction.
2. Select the Alcohol – High-proof vodka or brandy (40-50% alcohol) works best.
3. Combine in a Jar – Fill a glass jar with herbs and cover with alcohol.
4. Infuse for 4-6 Weeks - Store in a dark place, shaking occasionally.
5. Strain and Bottle—Remove plant material using cheesecloth or a fine sieve, then store in amber glass dropper bottles.

Non-Alcoholic Alternatives

- Glycerin Tinctures – These are Sweeter and ideal for children.
- Vinegar Tinctures – Used for culinary and medicinal applications.

Tinctures provide concentrated doses of herbs, making them a versatile addition to an herbalist's toolkit.

Salves and Balms: Herbal Healing for the Skin

Salves and balms represent a harmonious blend of herbal-infused oils and natural waxes, meticulously crafted to formulate topical remedies that relieve various skin ailments, including minor wounds, muscle aches, and various dermatological conditions. Start by carefully selecting herbs with known healing properties and infusing them into carrier oils like olive, coconut, or almond oil. This infusion process is pivotal, as it allows the therapeutic compounds of the herbs to be extracted and merged with the oil, creating a potent herbal concentrate. Once the herbs have imparted their essence into the oil, the mixture is gently heated with beeswax—or candelilla wax as a vegan alternative—to thicken it into a spreadable consistency. This step is crucial for formulating salves and balms, as it determines their texture and ease of application.

The choice of wax contributes to the final product's solidity and enhances its protective qualities, sealing in moisture and forming a barrier that supports the skin's natural healing processes. After achieving the desired consistency, the mixture is carefully poured into tins or glass jars and allowed to cool and solidify. This transformation culminates in a versatile and soothing remedy, ready to be applied directly to the skin. Lavender, for its calming and antibacterial properties; comfrey, renowned for its ability to heal bruises and sprains; and calendula, celebrated for its soothing effect on irritated skin, are among the popular choices for these preparations.

Salves and balms are essential to natural skin care, offering a gentle yet practical approach to treating and nurturing the skin. Through the thoughtful combination of herbal-infused oils and natural waxes, these remedies harness the potent healing power of nature, providing a direct and comforting application that supports the body's innate healing abilities. To develop your salves and balms, a summary of the steps is here:

- Infuse the Oil – Steep dried herbs in a carrier oil (olive, coconut, or almond) for several weeks.
- Strain and Heat—Warm the infused oil and add beeswax or candelilla wax to make a vegan alternative.
- Pour and Cool – Transfer to tins or glass jars and allow to solidify.

Lavender, comfrey, and calendula are popular soothing salves that promote skin healing and relaxation.

Herbal Poultices and Compresses: Direct Healing Applications

Poultices and compresses are dynamic methods of applying herbal remedies directly to the skin, targeting specific areas for immediate therapeutic effects. These applications are particularly effective in drawing out impurities, alleviating swelling, and calming irritated tissues.

Poultices are made by crushing fresh herbs into a thick paste, then spreading it directly onto the skin or placing it between two layers of cloth before application. This method ensures that the herbs' active constituents are in close contact with the affected area, promoting healing by directly absorbing the plant's beneficial properties. Poultices are especially useful for treating local inflammations, wounds, bites, and stings, as they help to draw out toxins, ease pain, and reduce swelling.

Compresses are made by soaking a clean cloth in a potent herbal infusion or decoction and then applying it to the skin. The warmth or coolness of the compress, depending on the treatment required, aids in the penetration of the herbal constituents, providing relief and accelerating the healing process. Compresses are ideal for broader areas of inflammation or discomfort, such as abdominal pain, muscle aches, or skin irritations. You can reapply them several times, which offers a gentle yet effective way to administer herbal remedies. Both poultices and compresses exemplify the traditional practice of applying herbal medicine directly to the body, allowing for targeted treatment that leverages the natural healing power of plants. This hands-on approach facilitates physical healing and fosters a deeper connection between the individual and the healing processes of nature. The basic steps for creating your poultices and compresses are listed here.

Poultices

1. Prepare Fresh Herbs – Mash into a paste using a mortar and pestle.
2. Apply to the Skin – Spread onto affected areas and cover with a clean cloth.

3. Secure and Rest – Leave in place for 20-30 minutes before rinsing.

Compresses

1. Brew a Strong Infusion – Soak a clean cloth in the warm herbal liquid.
2. Apply to the Body – Lay over the affected area and cover with a towel.
3. Reapply as needed – Repeat for 15-30 minutes for best results.

Common herbs for poultices and compresses include ginger (warming), arnica (anti-inflammatory), and plantain (wound healing).

Safety and Storage: Preserving Herbal Preparations

Ensuring the potency and longevity of herbal remedies is paramount, and you can achieve this through meticulous handling and storage practices. Labeling and dating each preparation meticulously immediately after production is crucial, as well as providing clear information on the contents and creation date. This step is essential not only for organization but also for tracking the shelf life of your remedies. Utilizing airtight containers is another critical measure. These containers keep out moisture and air, which can significantly compromise the quality of herbal preparations and maintain the integrity of the remedies. Maintaining the effectiveness of herbal products requires proper storage conditions.

A calm, dark environment is optimal, shielding the remedies from the deteriorating effects of light and heat. Sunlight, in particular, can degrade the active compounds in herbs, while excessive heat can cause oils to turn rancid and dry herbs to lose their potency more rapidly. "Keep a close eye on your stored herbal remedies to ensure they stay safe and effective. Indicators like mold growth, unpleasant odors, or discoloration signal that the product is unsafe. Following proper handling and storage guidelines can significantly extend the life of your herbal remedies, preserving their healing properties and ensuring they remain a potent and safe choice for wellness.

- Label and Date – Always mark jars with contents and preparation dates.
- Use Airtight Containers – Prevents contamination and preserves freshness.
- Store in a Cool, Dark Place – Light and heat degrade herbal compounds.
- Monitor for Spoilage – Discard any preparations with mold, off smells, or discoloration.

The Timeless Art of Herbal Medicine

Mastering herbal preparations is both a science and an art, blending tradition with personal exploration. Anyone can harness plants' healing power by understanding infusions, decoctions, tinctures, salves, and poultices. These time-honored techniques allow us to connect with nature, nurture our health, and pass down the wisdom of herbal medicine for generations to come.

In the next chapter, we will delve into the science of herbal Medicine, and how plants support the body's natural healing, exploring their impact on the body. Let's continue our journey into the heart of nature's healing remedies.🌿✨

The Science of Herbal Medicine: How Plants Support the Body's Natural Healing

For centuries, herbal medicine has been pivotal in holistic wellness, offering natural remedies that work harmoniously with the body's physiological processes. The **human body and medicinal plants** share an intricate relationship, where bioactive compounds in herbs interact with different organs, promoting balance, healing, and vitality.

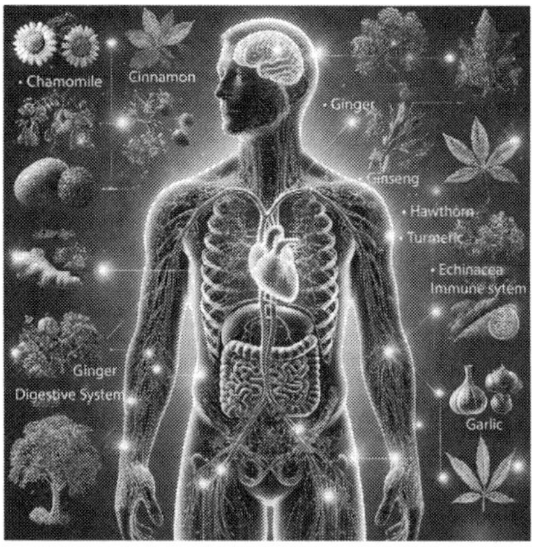

This detailed illustration captures the essence of **herbal synergy**, mapping the connection between key herbs and the body systems they support.

Unlocking the Healing Power of Nature

This representation shows **organ-herb pairings** to enhance understanding of how specific plants support human health. These pairings illustrate how herbal medicine is not just about symptom relief but **restoring equilibrium in the body** by addressing root causes.

Energy Flow Representation: The Path of Herbal Absorption

One of the most striking features of this illustration is the **glowing energy pathways** flowing through the veins and vital organs. This visual effect represents the **bioavailability** of herbal compounds—the journey of medicinal plant constituents through the body. When herbs are ingested, their **phytochemicals** (plant-based active compounds) go through the following stages:

1. **Absorption** – Herbal constituents are absorbed through the digestive tract, entering the bloodstream.
2. **Metabolism & Distribution** – These compounds travel through the circulatory system, targeting specific organs or tissues based on their properties.
3. **Cellular Utilization** – The body uses these compounds to heal, nourish, and regulate biochemical functions.
4. **Detoxification & Elimination** – The liver and kidneys process and excrete unneeded compounds, ensuring a balanced system.

This visualization's **glowing veins and illuminated organs** highlight this dynamic energy exchange, reinforcing how plant-based medicine integrates seamlessly with bodily processes.

Key Herb-Organ Pairings in the Illustration

Each herb in this depiction **supports specific organs and systems**, contributing to overall wellness. Below is a breakdown of the essential **herb-organ pairings** and their corresponding benefits:

- **Chamomile (Matricaria chamomilla) for the Brain & Nervous System** – Known for its calming properties, chamomile soothes anxiety, supports sleep, and reduces nervous tension.
- **Echinacea (Echinacea purpurea) for the Immune System** – A powerful immune booster, echinacea enhances the body's defenses and reduces the severity of colds and infections.
- **Ginger (Zingiber officinale) for Digestion & Circulation** – A natural digestive aid, ginger alleviates nausea, stimulates circulation and supports metabolic function.
- **Garlic (Allium sativum) for the Liver & Cardiovascular System** – Renowned for its detoxifying effects, garlic supports liver function, reduces cholesterol, and promotes heart health.
- **Hawthorn (Crataegus monogyna) for the Heart** – Strengthens the heart muscle, enhances circulation, and regulates blood pressure.
- **Turmeric (Curcuma longa) for Inflammation & Joints** – Reduces inflammation, protects against oxidative stress, and supports joint mobility.
- **Ginseng (Panax ginseng) for Energy & Stamina** – Boosts energy, enhances cognitive function and supports adrenal health.

Each of these herbs contributes **to symptom relief and restoring systemic balance**, ensuring long-term health benefits.

A Holistic Perspective on Herbal Healing

The charm of herbal medicine is found in its **holistic approach**—rather than targeting isolated symptoms, it **nourishes, balances, and**

restores the body as a whole. This illustration is a visual guide to comprehending how herbs support key organs, emphasizing **the interconnectedness of nature and human health**.

By integrating the wisdom of herbal traditions with the advancements in contemporary science, we can harness the potential of medicinal plants, empowering individuals to take charge of their health naturally. Whether using herbs for **preventative care, targeted healing, or overall vitality**, their ability to work **in sync with the body's innate healing mechanisms** makes them a powerful tool in holistic wellness.

Your journey into **natural healing** starts here—embracing the timeless wisdom of herbal medicine to promote **vibrancy, balance, and well-being**.

As we've explored, herbal medicine aligns with the body's natural rhythms—supporting digestion, enhancing immunity, reducing inflammation, and restoring balance. With a deeper understanding of how herbs interact with the body, the next step is discovering the plants.

The following section explores individual herb profiles, detailing their traditional uses, scientific benefits, and how we can incorporate herbs into daily life. Whether seeking gentle support for overall wellness or targeted remedies for specific concerns, these time-honored plants hold the key to holistic healing. 🌿✨

Herb Profiles and Their Uses

"Embrace the power of natural remedies to build resilience, combat stress, and support holistic wellness."

Imagine a time when the world felt chaotic, and your mind was a whirlwind of thoughts. In those moments, the gentle power of adaptogens can be a lifeline. These remarkable herbs, with a history dating back to the work of Russian scientist N. Lazarev in 1940, offer a natural way to bolster resilience against life's stresses. The concept of adaptogens, further refined by researchers like I. Brekhman and Dardymov, is that they are natural substances that help maintain homeostasis and support the immune-neuro-endocrine system.

Adaptogens ensure that our bodily systems operate smoothly, even in stressful situations. They interact with the hypothalamic–pituitary–adrenal (HPA) axis, a complex system involving the interaction between the hypothalamus, pituitary gland, and adrenal glands. They play a critical role in the body's response to stress. Adaptogens help regulate stress hormones like cortisol, enabling the body to respond more effectively to challenges. The result is a more resilient system, capable of withstanding stress without succumbing to fatigue or illness.

Ashwagandha, a plant from India and parts of Africa, is known to calm the mind and reduce anxiety. Research shows that it has a positive impact on anxiety and stress. Compounds like withanolides in this herb produce calming effects, helping lower cortisol levels and promoting well-being. As you incorporate Ashwagandha into your routine, you'll likely notice a newfound sense of calm, allowing you to navigate life's storms with grace and composure.

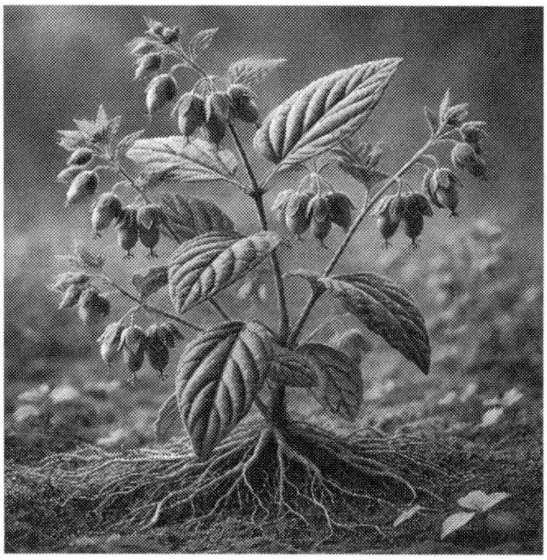

A detailed botanical illustration of an Ashwagandha plant (Withania somnifera) is here. The image highlights its green leaves, small yellowish flowers, and distinctive red berries, representing its traditional herbal medicine use.

Rhodiola, a powerful adaptogen, is well-known for its capacity to boost mental clarity and reduce fatigue. Often used by Russian cosmonauts and athletes to improve performance, Rhodiola has a long history of use in traditional medicine. This herb effectively reduces mental fatigue and improves cognitive function, making it an invaluable ally during intense mental exertion. Scientific studies support these claims, revealing that Rhodiola can improve attention, accuracy, and overall cognitive performance. Its active compounds, such as rosavin and salidroside, positively impact mood and mental acuity.

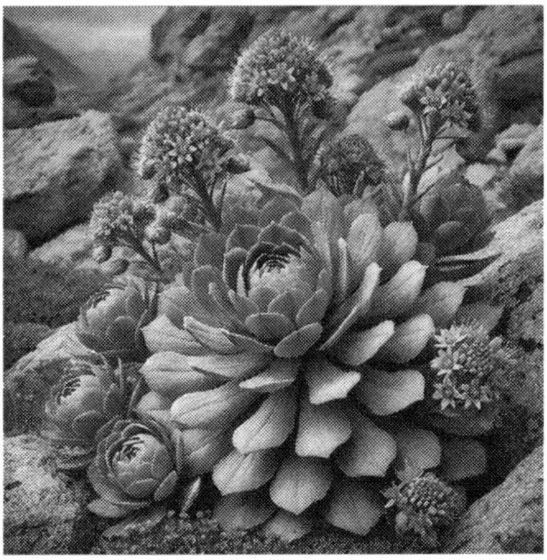

Here is a detailed botanical illustration of a **Rhodiola plant (Rhodiola rosea)**. The image highlights its **thick, succulent-like green leaves, clusters of small yellowish flowers, and sturdy roots**, representing its traditional use in herbal medicine to enhance resilience and vitality.

Holy basil, or tulsi, is another adaptogen with deep cultural roots, particularly in India, where it is considered a sacred plant. This herb is renowned for balancing cortisol levels and supporting the body's response to stress. Holy basil's adaptogenic properties are complemented by its antioxidant and anti-inflammatory effects, making it a versatile herb for promoting overall health. In traditional Ayurvedic practices, holy basil enhances mental clarity and supports the immune system, allowing individuals to maintain resilience in the face of stress. Modern research validates these uses, showing that holy basil can help modulate stress responses and improve mental function.

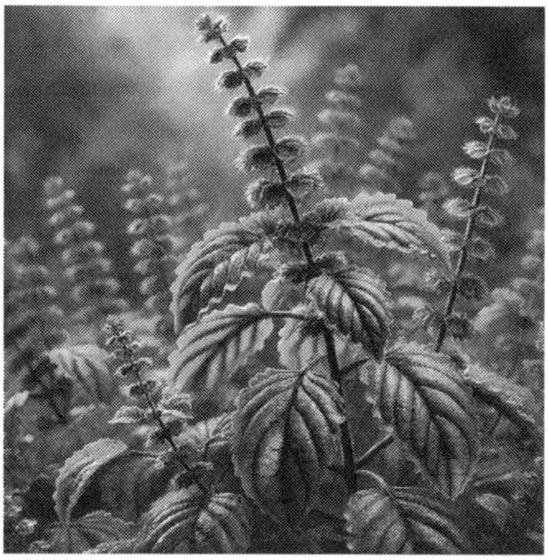

Here is a detailed botanical illustration of a **Holy Basil (Tulsi) plant**. The image features **vibrant green leaves, delicate purple flowers, and slender stems**, highlighting its **medicinal and spiritual significance** in herbal medicine and Ayurveda.

Adaptogens are unique to traditional medicine systems such as Ayurveda and Traditional Chinese Medicine (TCM). They often balance the body's energy and support overall vitality.

Studies, such as those conducted by Frontiers in Pharmacology, US Department of Veterans Affairs Whole Health Library, and Dr. Tieraona Low Dog, have shown that adaptogens can enhance cellular energy, improve sleep, and support recovery from stress. Their ability to stabilize the neuroendocrine system and optimize the body's response to stress makes them invaluable allies in our fast-paced world. As you explore the world of adaptogens, you'll discover a rich tapestry of herbs, each with unique properties and benefits. These remarkable plants invite you to cultivate resilience and embrace a life of balance and vitality.

ANTIMICROBIALS: HERBAL ALLIES FOR IMMUNE SUPPORT

Consider the world of microorganisms, unseen yet omnipresent, constantly interacting with our bodies. Here lies the vital role of herbal antimicrobials, nature's defenders against pathogens such as bacteria, viruses, and fungi. These herbs bolster our immune systems, providing a natural shield that protects and supports our health. Antimicrobial herbs work through various mechanisms. They disrupt bacterial cell walls, inhibiting their growth. They may inhibit viral replication, stopping infections in their tracks. Some even enhance the body's natural defenses, stimulating the immune system to fight off invaders more effectively.

Echinacea stands out among these antimicrobial herbs, renowned for its ability to reduce cold symptoms and support the immune system. This North American plant has been used for centuries by indigenous tribes, who recognized its power to fend off infections. Modern science has validated these traditional uses and enhanced our understanding of its mechanisms, with studies showing that echinacea can reduce the severity and duration of colds.

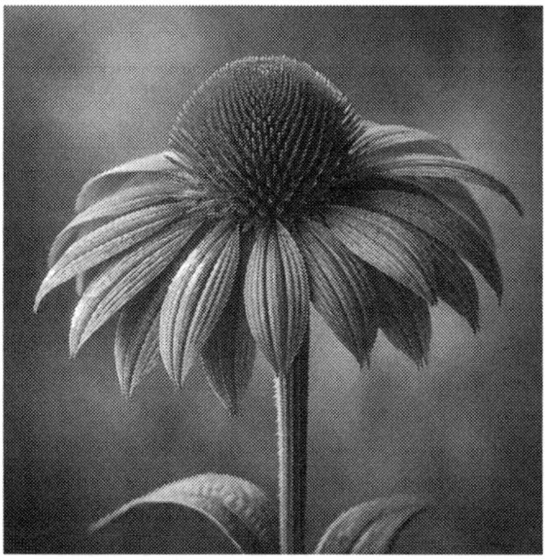

Here is a detailed botanical illustration of an **Echinacea plant (Echinacea purpurea)**. The image highlights its **vibrant pinkish-purple petals, spiky orange-brown central cone, and sturdy green leaves**, representing its traditional use in herbal medicine for immune support.

Garlic, with its unmistakable pungent aroma, is another potent antimicrobial herb. "People across cultures and centuries have used this herb in folk medicine, often hailing it as a natural antibiotic. Garlic's active compound, allicin, prevents harmful bacteria growth, making it an effective infection remedy. Beyond its antibacterial prowess, garlic also boasts antiviral and antifungal activities, making it a versatile and comprehensive addition to your herbal toolkit.

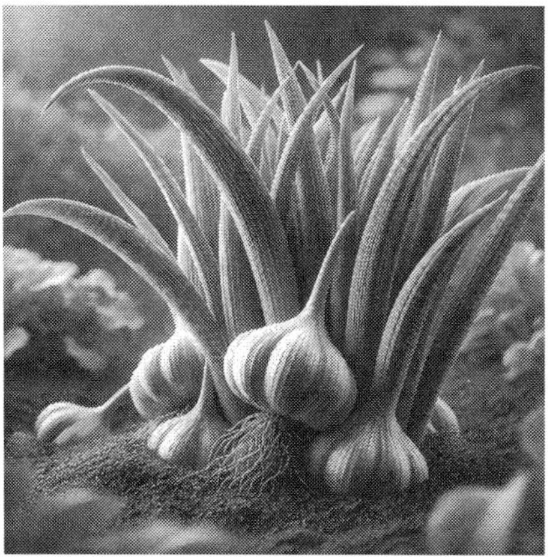

Here is a detailed botanical illustration of a **Garlic plant (Allium sativum)**. The image highlights its **long, slender green leaves, a bulb with multiple cloves partially exposed in the soil, and delicate white-pink flowers atop a tall stalk**, emphasizing its culinary and medicinal importance.

Several people celebrate Elderberry for its antiviral support, particularly during flu season. This dark, berry-laden shrub has been a staple in European herbal medicine for generations. Elderberry's rich anthocyanins provide its deep color and potent health benefits. These compounds interfere with the flu virus's ability to enter cells, effectively reducing the duration and severity of symptoms. Elderberry syrup, a modern adaptation of this traditional remedy, has become a popular supplement for boosting immunity and warding off seasonal illnesses. It's sweet, tangy flavor makes it a favorite among children and adults, offering a palatable way to support health naturally.

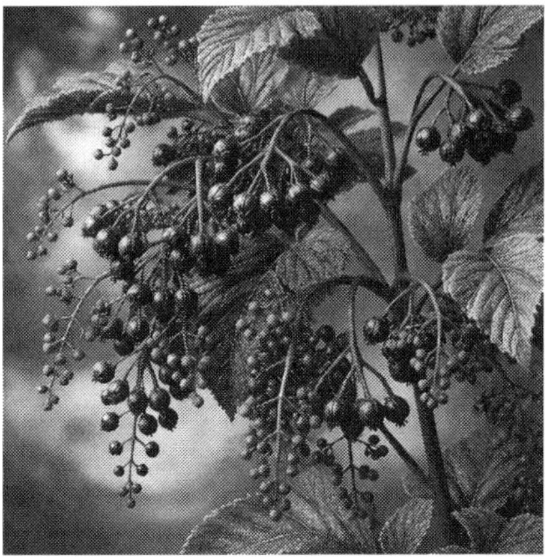

Here is a detailed botanical illustration of an **Elderberry plant (Sambucus nigra)**. The image highlights **clusters of deep purple-black berries, delicate white flower clusters, and serrated green leaves**, emphasizing its medicinal and immune-boosting properties.

The applications of antimicrobial herbs are as diverse as their histories. Garlic, for instance, has been used in traditional medicine as a remedy for respiratory infections and digestive issues. Its ability to enhance circulation and improve heart health has also made it a staple in folk remedies. In contemporary settings, garlic is often found in supplements, providing a concentrated dose of allicin without needing fresh cloves. With its antiviral properties, Elderberry has found a new niche as a modern supplement. Elderberry syrup is a convenient way to incorporate this powerful herb into daily routines, offering a sweet defense against colds and flu.

While antimicrobial herbs offer numerous benefits, using them safely and wisely is essential. Echinacea, for example, is most effective when taken at the first sign of a cold. A typical dosage might involve 300 to 500 milligrams of dried root or 2.5 milliliters of tincture taken thrice daily. Please do not use it long-term, as its efficacy decreases over time. Garlic, though generally safe, can interact with certain medications, particularly blood thinners.

Nervines: Calming Herbs for Mental Well-Being

Imagine winding down after a long day, your body weary and your mind racing. In this situation, you can use the herb nerves, which can offer a gentle hand to soothe your nervous system and nurture mental wellness. These herbal allies interact with neurotransmitters—chemical messengers in your brain that influence mood and stress response—to foster relaxation and tranquility. Through their calming effects on the central nervous system, nerves help ease anxiety, promote restful sleep, and uplift the spirit, allowing you to navigate life's challenges with a steadier mind.

Valerian is among the most revered nervines, often likened to nature's lullaby. This herb's sedative properties help combat insomnia and anxiety. Valerenic acid in valerian interacts with brain gamma-aminobutyric acid (GABA) receptors, producing its calming effects. These receptors play a key role in promoting relaxation and reducing nerve excitability. By enhancing the activity of GABA, valerian induces a sense of calm, making it easier to drift into slumber. Whether used as a tincture, capsule, or tea, valerian can be a comforting addition to your nighttime routine, gently coaxing your body into restfulness.

Chamomile, shown earlier with the 25 Herbs in Chapter 2, is another beloved nervine known for easing anxiety and tension with its delicate daisy-like blooms. This herb has been cherished for centuries in European traditions, often steeped into a warm, soothing tea. Chamomile's calming effects are mainly due to apigenin, which mimics the action of prescription sedatives, albeit in a much milder, natural form. Regularly sipping chamomile tea can help relax your muscles, quiet your mind, and prepare you for a tranquil night's sleep.

With its refreshing citrus scent, Lemon balm is a nervine or herb known to address anxiety and nervousness by calming, soothing, uplifting, and invigorating. Lemon balm, shown earlier with the 25 Herbs in Chapter 2, frequently used to boost mood and cognitive function, can be a powerful ally in combating stress and anxiety. This herb contains rosmarinic acid, which increases the availability of GABA in the brain, much like valerian. This boost in GABA activity helps stabilize your mood and reduce feelings of nervousness. Lemon balm's versatile nature makes it an easy addition to your daily life, providing a subtle yet effective way to support mental well-being.

Throughout history, nerves have played a vital role in cultural healing practices. In European herbal traditions, Chamomile was often used in rituals to promote peace and relaxation, reflecting its deep-rooted significance as a calming herb. Healers believed Chamomile helped to ward off nightmares and bring restful sleep. Similarly, Greek and Roman healers cherished lemon balm for its mood-enhancing properties. These historical uses highlight the timeless appeal of nervines as natural remedies for mental distress, underscoring their enduring relevance in today's fast-paced world.

Incorporating nervousness into your daily routine can be a delightful and rewarding practice. Chamomile tea, for instance, is a simple yet effective way to unwind in the evening.

Digestive Aids: Herbs for a Healthy Gut

Visualize your gut as a vibrant ecosystem complete with life and activity. Our gut's inner world is crucial and is known to have a far-reaching effect on our bodies. When this system falls out of balance, discomfort and digestive issues can arise, impacting your well-being. Fortunately, nature provides a bounty of herbs to support and restore digestive health, relieving common ailments.

One of the most celebrated digestive aids is ginger. People have used this knobby root, with its warm, spicy aroma, for centuries to soothe nausea and settle upset stomachs. Its active compounds, including gingerols and shogaols, have anti-inflammatory properties, which help relax the gastrointestinal tract. In Ayurvedic medicine, people revere ginger for its digestive fire, or "agni," believed to enhance digestion and assimilation of nutrients. You can add ginger to your daily life by brewing simple ginger tea. Just slice fresh ginger root, steep it in boiling water, and sip slowly. This warming infusion eases nausea and supports digestion during pregnancy, travel, or illness.

Peppermint, with its refreshing scent, is another powerhouse for digestive health. Known for its ability to soothe irritable bowel syndrome (IBS), Peppermint relaxes the muscles of the gastrointestinal tract, reducing spasms and discomfort. Its menthol content is responsible for this calming effect, making peppermint oil capsules convenient for those seeking relief. These capsules can ease symptoms like bloating, gas, and abdominal pain, providing a cooling sensation that eases digestive distress. Take a capsule before meals to help manage IBS symptoms and promote smooth digestion.

Fennel's delicate, feathery fronds offer a gentle touch to digestive troubles. This aromatic herb, a favorite in many cultures, reduces bloating and gas.

Across the globe, different cultures have harnessed the power of these herbs to support digestion. In Ayurvedic practices, ginger is a staple, often included in teas and recipes to enhance flavor and aid digestion. Its warming properties make it a perfect addition to curries and soups, where it adds zest and supports the digestive process. Peppermint has been used in European and Middle Eastern traditions to flavor teas and confections, offering taste and digestive benefits. Fennel, too, has found its way into culinary traditions worldwide, from Italian sausages to Indian spice blends, each use rooted in its digestive prowess.

Adding these herbs to your daily meals and remedies can be a straightforward yet transformative practice.

Circulatory Boosters: Herbs for Heart Health

In the gentle rhythm of a heartbeat lies the essence of life, a pulse that carries vitality through every vein. Herbs that support circulatory health work harmoniously with this natural rhythm, enhancing cardiovascular wellness. These herbs are nature's allies in maintaining a healthy heart and robust circulation, offering a holistic approach to cardiovascular care. Promoting better circulation ensures oxygen and nutrients reach every cell, supporting overall health and vitality. They also help protect the delicate lining of blood vessels and promote smooth, efficient blood movement.

. . .

Hawthorn is a herb that supports heart health. This small, thorny shrub has been vital in European herbal medicine for centuries, often used to support heart function and manage blood pressure. It emphasizes its traditional use in herbal medicine for heart health and circulation support.

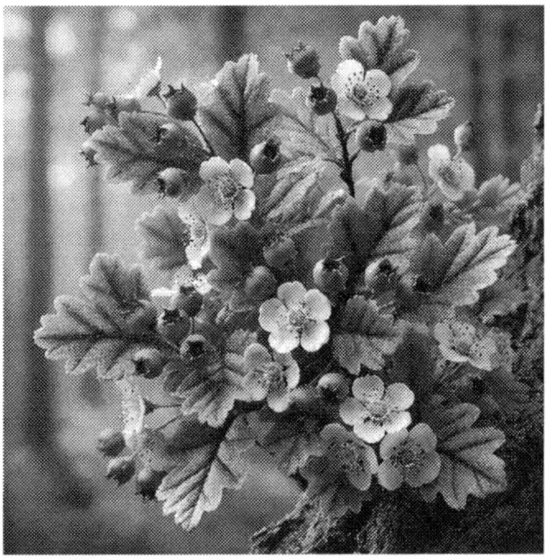

With its fiery heat, Cayenne, which I love, is another powerful herb that stimulates circulation and invigorates the cardiovascular system. The active compound in Cayenne, capsaicin, helps to keep blood pressure down and reduce the risk of clot formation. Beyond its circulatory benefits, Cayenne aids digestion, promotes metabolism, and provides a warming, invigorating energy that can enhance physical performance. Whether used in cooking or as a supplement, Cayenne offers a versatile and dynamic way to support heart health and vitality.

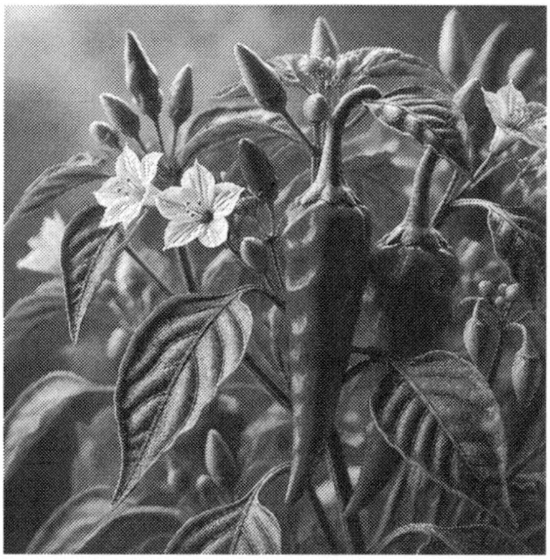

Here is a detailed botanical illustration of a **Cayenne Pepper plant (Capsicum annuum)**. The image highlights **vibrant red chili peppers hanging from green stems, ovate dark green leaves, and small white star-shaped flowers**, emphasizing its culinary and medicinal uses for boosting circulation and metabolism.

Ginkgo biloba, known for its distinctive fan-shaped leaves, supports cognitive functions. This ancient tree, often considered a living fossil in China, improves blood flow in the brain and other extremities. Ginkgo's active compounds, including flavonoids and terpenoids, help protect blood vessels and improve peripheral circulation, making it a valuable herb for those experiencing cold hands and feet or age-related cognitive decline. Research indicates that ginkgo improves memory, attention, and overall cognitive function, aiding mental clarity and focus as you age.

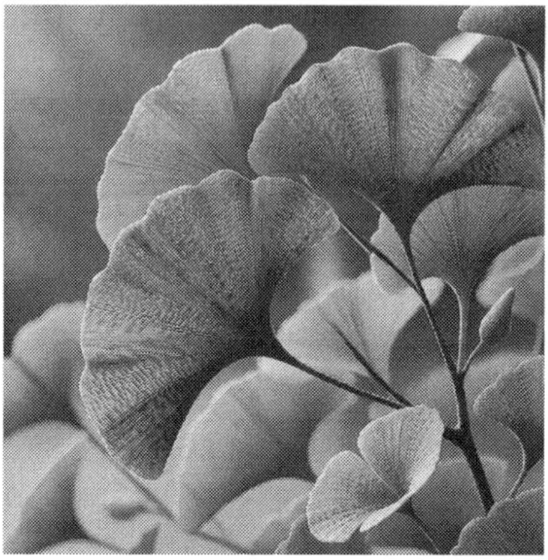

Here is a detailed botanical illustration of a **Ginkgo biloba tree**. The image highlights its **distinctive fan-shaped green leaves with delicate veins, some turning golden yellow in autumn**, emphasizing its traditional medicinal use for cognitive support and circulation.

In European traditions, hawthorn was often used in rituals to symbolize love and protection, reflecting its role in safeguarding the heart. Indigenous cultures in the Americas have long used Cayenne to stimulate circulation and boost energy, highlighting its rich history. The Indigenous culture saw Cayenne's vibrant red color and fiery heat as symbols of vitality and strength. Ginkgo biloba, with its ancient lineage, has been revered in Chinese culture for millennia, often planted in temple gardens as a symbol of longevity and resilience.

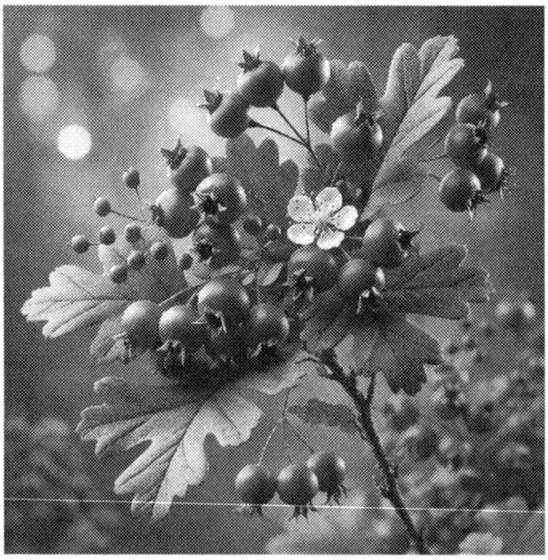

Here is a detailed botanical illustration of a **Hawthorn plant (Crataegus monogyna)**. The image highlights **serrated green leaves, clusters of small white flowers with pink stamens, and bright red berries growing on thorny branches**. It emphasizes its traditional use in herbal medicine for heart health and circulation support.

Studies have found that ginkgo can improve symptoms of intermittent claudication, a condition characterized by poor leg circulation. Similarly, studies on Cayenne have demonstrated its ability to help blood flow. By exploring the rich tapestry of circulatory herbs, you can integrate these powerful allies into your daily routine, supporting a healthy heart and vibrant life.

Skin Saviors: Herbs for Topical and Internal Use

Imagine your skin as a mirror, reflecting the health and vitality within. Herbs' role in skincare is diverse and profound, offering solutions that work from the outside and the inside. When applied topically, herbs can reduce inflammation, soothe irritation, and promote healing. Internally, they support detoxification, nourish tissues, and enhance the body's natural regenerative processes. This dual action makes herbs versatile and a good ally for seeking healthy, radiant skin.

Calendula, with its bright orange petals, is a quintessential skin-supporting herb. "People know this herb for its remarkable ability to heal wounds and have used it in folk medicine for centuries to treat cuts, scrapes, and minor burns.

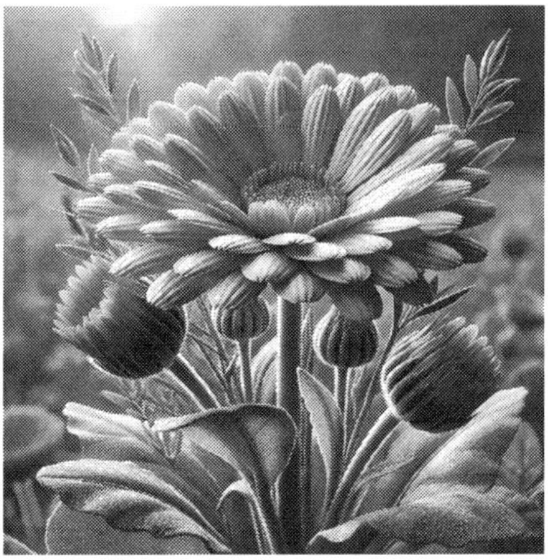

Here is a detailed botanical illustration of a **Calendula plant (Calendula officinalis)**. The image highlights its **vibrant orange and yellow daisy-like flowers, delicate petals, and green lance-shaped leaves**, emphasizing its traditional use in herbal medicine for skin healing and anti-inflammatory benefits.

Aloe vera is another powerhouse in skin care. It's packed with vitamins and minerals, providing a soothing balm for burns and sun-damaged skin. The ancient Egyptians revered aloe vera for its beauty-enhancing properties, incorporating it into their daily rituals. Modern studies have confirmed aloe's efficacy in reducing inflammation and promoting skin regeneration, making it a staple in many skincare products.

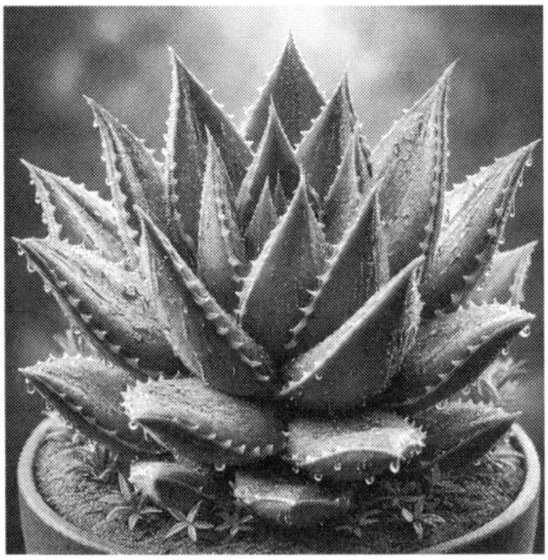

Here is a detailed botanical illustration of an **Aloe vera plant (Aloe barbadensis miller)**. The image highlights **thick, fleshy green leaves with serrated edges arranged in a rosette pattern. A cross-section reveals the translucent gel inside**, emphasizing its traditional use for skin healing, hydration, and medicinal benefits.

Burdock root, though less commonly known, is vital in detoxifying the skin. Burdock helps cleanse the bloodstream and eliminate toxins. This internal purification can lead to more precise, healthier skin, free from blemishes and irritation. You support your body's natural detox processes by incorporating burdock root into your diet, whether as a tea or supplement. This holistic approach to skincare addresses the root causes of skin issues, promoting balance and vitality from the inside out.

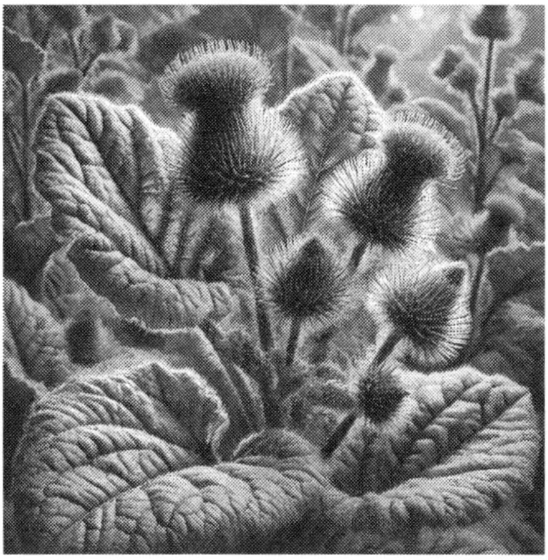

Here is a detailed botanical illustration of a **Burdock plant (Arctium lappa)**. The image highlights **large, broad green leaves with wavy edges, tall purple thistle-like flowers, and long, thick roots partially exposed in the soil**. It emphasizes its traditional use in herbal medicine for detoxification and skin health.

The evolution of herbal skincare reflects a rich tapestry of history and innovation. Aloe Vera's ancient use in Egyptian beauty rituals highlights the timeless appeal of natural remedies. These traditions have been passed down through generations, evolving into modern applications that blend past wisdom with contemporary science.

Creating your herbal skincare products can be a great experience. A simple calendula-infused oil, as mentioned earlier, is a great starting point. Combine fresh aloe gel with a few drops of vitamin E oil and a dash of lavender essential oil for a soothing aloe vera gel. This blend not only cools and hydrates but also provides antioxidant protection, supporting your skin's health and resilience by experimenting with different herbs and formulations, looking at your unique needs, and embracing the natural beauty of herbs in every application.

In our exploration of skin-supporting herbs, we've uncovered how these natural remedies offer topical and internal benefits. As you integrate these herbs into your routine, you'll find they enhance your skin's appearance and contribute to your overall well-being. With the knowledge and tools to harness the power of nature, you're well-equipped to nurture your skin and embrace a healthier, more radiant you.

As we explore the world of herbal remedies, it becomes clear that every plant has specific characteristics and benefits that can contribute to various areas of our health. From the stress-balancing power of adaptogens to the antimicrobial benefits of herbal allies, nature provides a diverse pharmacy waiting to be understood and utilized.

However, knowledge of herbs alone is only part of the journey. Understanding how to **integrate these remedies into daily life** practically and effectively is just as crucial. In the next chapter, we will move beyond theory and into action—exploring **how to incorporate herbal remedies seamlessly into your routine**.

In **Chapter 6: Integrating Herbal Remedies into Daily Life**, we'll delve into strategies for making herbal healing a natural part of your lifestyle. Whether through simple teas, tinctures, or culinary infusions, you'll learn how to harness the power of herbs effortlessly in your everyday routine. Get ready to bring the wisdom of herbal medicine into your daily practice, making wellness an ongoing, enjoyable experience. 🌿✨

Integrating Herbal Remedies into Daily Life

"Seamlessly integrate the healing power of herbs into your daily routine for effortless, holistic wellness."

Picture a bustling kitchen on a weekday morning, the air filled with the aroma of freshly brewed coffee and the soft hum of a blender. Amidst the chaos of getting ready for the day, you find a moment to pause and add a spoonful of adaptogenic herbs to your smoothie. This simple act, woven seamlessly into your daily routine, is a testament to the power of herbal remedies to enhance your life without demanding more of your time. In our fast-paced world, where every minute counts, integrating herbal practices into your lifestyle can provide profound benefits without requiring painstaking effort. This chapter will examine how we can effectively incorporate these natural allies into our daily lives.

Herbal Remedies for Busy Lifestyles: Simple and Accessible Solutions

Time-efficient herbal practices offer an effortless way to bring herbal medicine into your routine. Consider the simplicity of herbal teas that brew in minutes, transforming boiling water and a handful of dried herbs into a soothing cup of wellness. Chamomile or peppermint teas, for instance, provide calming effects and can be easily prepared as you go about your morning tasks. These teas deliver immediate benefits and create a comforting ritual, encouraging mindfulness amidst the morning rush. The ease and convenience of these practices can help you feel empowered and in control of your health, even in the busiest of times.

For those on the move, ready-made tinctures are invaluable allies. Compact and potent, they offer the convenience of on-the-go use, ensuring that the therapeutic benefits of herbs are always within reach. Whether you seek the calming embrace of lavender or the immune-boosting power of echinacea, a few drops under the tongue or in a glass of water can serve as a quick, effective remedy. Keeping these tinctures in your bag or desk drawer allows you to seamlessly integrate their use into your daily rhythm, enhancing your well-being without disrupting your schedule.

Multitasking with herbal remedies can maximize your time efficiency, turning ordinary routines into opportunities for healing. Imagine the invigorating start to your day when you blend adaptogens like ashwagandha into your morning smoothie. These herbs bolster your resilience against stress, equipping you to face the day calmly and focus. Similarly, incorporating essential oils into your bath can help make that bath a refreshing adventure. The aromatic compounds of eucalyptus or lavender permeate the steam, offering respiratory relief and promoting relaxation. By layering these practices over existing routines, you weave the benefits of herbs into the fabric of daily life, feeling flexible and adaptable in your health practices.

Overnight infusions are ideal for those seeking quick and easy herbal preparations. Before bed, place your chosen herbs in a jar of water and allow them to steep overnight. In the morning, strain the liquid and enjoy a refreshing herbal infusion to start your day. This method requires minimal effort and provides a gentle, sustained release of herbal benefits.

Staying the course and repeating the process is essential to changing your life and focusing on herbal remedies, even in a busy lifestyle.

Setting reminders for herbal dosage can help you establish regular use, ensuring that you don't miss out on their cumulative effects. Digital tools or simple sticky notes prompt you to take tinctures or prepare teas. Keeping herbs accessible in common areas, like the kitchen counter or bathroom shelf, further enhances consistency. When herbs are within easy reach, they allow you to turn intentions into habits.

Interactive Element: Herbal Routine Checklist

- Identify and select a few herbs that align with your wellness goals.
- Designate a specific time or activity where you can integrate herbal use.
- Keep tinctures and teas visible and accessible in your living space.
- Reflect on the effects and adjust your routine for optimal benefits.

Incorporating herbal remedies into a busy lifestyle is not about adding complexity but enhancing what you already do. By choosing simple, effective practices that fit effortlessly into your day, you unlock the potential of herbs to nurture and support you, even amidst the demands of modern life. This simplicity can make you feel at ease and confident in your health choices.

Balancing Herbal Remedies with Conventional Medicine

Integrating herbal remedies with conventional medicine offers opportunities and challenges in modern healthcare. It's essential to consult your doctor before making significant changes to your daily routine. This crucial step can reassure you and make you confident in your decisions.

When discussing herbal remedies, preparing a comprehensive list of all current herbal and pharmaceutical uses is helpful. This list should include not only the names of the herbs and medications but also their dosages and frequencies of use. Sharing this information equips your healthcare provider with the knowledge to offer tailored advice. It also fosters trust, demonstrating your commitment to a holistic, safe approach to wellness. Be open about your health goals and concerns and remember that your healthcare provider is your ally in achieving optimal health.

Understanding potential interactions between herbal remedies and conventional medicine is crucial. Some herbs can influence blood pressure and should be used cautiously with hypertension medications. For instance, St. John's Wort, which is known for its mood-enhancing properties, can interfere with the effectiveness of certain antidepressants and other drugs. Knowing these interactions, you can decide which herbs to include in your health regimen. It is also essential to monitor how your body responds to new treatment combinations and to consult your healthcare provider if you experience any adverse effects. Careful attention is necessary to maintain a safe and effective health plan, ensuring you feel secure and confident in your health choices.

Real-world examples can inspire and guide those looking to combine herbal and conventional treatments. Take the case of Jessica; for instance, Jessica experienced chronic migraines, and prescription medication only partially managed her condition. After consulting her doctor, she began incorporating feverfew and magnesium supplements into her routine. Over time, she noticed a decrease in both the frequency and intensity of her migraines, which allowed her to rely less on pharmaceuticals.

Jessica is experiencing relief from her migraines after incorporating feverfew and magnesium supplements into her routine.

Another example is Thomas, who dealt with high blood pressure. By working closely with his healthcare provider, he successfully added garlic supplements to his diet and his prescribed medication. This combination helped him achieve better blood pressure control and improved his overall cardiovascular health.

Thomas managed his high blood pressure with garlic supplements and prescribed medication.

These stories highlight the potential for herbal and conventional treatments to work together, enhancing each other's benefits while reducing reliance on medication. This realization can make you feel hopeful about your health journey. However, achieving these successes takes time. Each individual's journey is unique; what works for one person may not be suitable for another. Therefore, it's essential to approach this integration with an open mind and a readiness to learn from your experiences. Doing so can create a personalized health plan that aligns with your values and supports your long-term well-being.

Overcoming Time Constraints: Efficient Herbal Practices

Finding time to incorporate herbal remedies into our daily lives can seem overwhelming. Yet, with some planning and the proper techniques, you can streamline your herbal practices to fit even the busiest schedules. One effective method is batch-preparing tinctures and oils. This approach saves time and allows you to experiment with different blends, tailoring your preparations to meet the varied needs of your household. Once prepared, these tinctures require minimal daily attention, offering a quick and potent means of accessing herbal benefits.

Another time-saving technique involves using slow cookers for herbal infusions. Slow cookers provide a convenient way to extract the therapeutic properties of herbs without constant supervision. Add your herbs and water to the cooker, set it on low, and let it work its magic while you go about your day. This gentle, sustained heat ensures maximum extraction, resulting in rich, flavorful infusions ready for use when needed. Incorporating these methods into your routine makes herbal preparation an effortless part of your lifestyle, enabling you to enjoy the benefits of herbs without compromising time or convenience.

Apps dedicated to tracking herbal use and effects can be invaluable allies. They help you monitor your herb intake, note any reactions, and adjust dosages as needed. These digital logs provide a comprehensive view of your herbal practices, empowering you to make informed decisions about your health. Many apps offer reminders and alerts, ensuring you never miss a dose or preparation time. By leveraging these digital resources, you gain greater control and oversight of your herbal regimen, allowing you to integrate natural remedies into your life quickly and precisely.

Organizing your herbal supplies is another key aspect of efficient herbal practices. By creating a system for labeling and categorizing your herbs, you streamline selecting and using them. Consider grouping herbs by their therapeutic use, such as digestive aids, stress relievers, or immune boosters. This categorization simplifies finding the right herb for the right situation, reducing the time spent searching and increasing the time spent benefiting. Labeling each jar with the herb name, date of purchase, and source provides clarity. It ensures freshness, helping you maintain a well-organized and effective herbal collection that is easy to navigate and use.

Planning and scheduling are potent tools for overcoming time constraints and ensuring regular herbal practice. By setting specific times for herbal self-care, you create a consistent routine that becomes as natural as brushing your teeth. Whether dedicating a few minutes in the morning for a calming infusion or setting aside time in the evening for a restorative herbal bath, these scheduled moments of self-care become anchors in your day, providing stability and balance. Incorporating these practices into your daily planner elevates their importance, turning them into non-negotiable appointments that align with your well-being. Through thoughtful planning, you transform herbal practices from an occasional luxury into a regular, integral part of daily life.

Herbal First Aid: Essential Remedies for Common Ailments

Imagine you're outdoors, perhaps on a hike or enjoying a day at the park when a minor mishap occurs. A scrape from a fall or the sting of an insect bite can swiftly ruin your day. Fortunately, the wisdom of herbal first aid offers a natural and effective remedy. Assembling a herbal first aid kit is a proactive step towards self-sufficiency in handling everyday health issues. A calendula salve is one of the most versatile components of such a kit. Its anti-inflammatory and antimicrobial qualities promote rapid healing while reducing the risk of infection.

Lavender oil is another essential addition, perfect for treating minor burns and soothing irritated skin. These easily prepared and stored remedies offer a natural alternative to commercial products, aligning with a holistic approach to health and well-being.

Quick-response herbal treatments are invaluable for common ailments, offering immediate relief with minimal preparation. Take peppermint tea, a simple yet effective remedy for headaches. A steaming cup of freshly brewed peppermint tea provides soothing relief and a refreshing addition to your routine. For motion sickness, ginger is a time-honored remedy. Its anti-inflammatory properties and ability to settle the stomach make it an excellent choice for nausea and digestive discomfort. A piece of candied ginger or ginger tea can work wonders, providing comfort and stability when moving.

Creating first aid preparations at home is straightforward, allowing you to tailor remedies to your needs. A comfrey poultice is particularly effective for sprains or bruises, drawing on comfrey's renowned ability to support tissue repair and reduce swelling. Comfrey is a perennial herb known for its medicinal properties. To make a poultice, crush fresh comfrey leaves into a paste, then apply it to the affected area, securing it with a clean cloth. This application accelerates recovery by promoting cell regeneration and reducing inflammation. Thoughtfully prepared, these preparations empower you to naturally and effectively manage minor injuries.

While herbal remedies offer significant benefits, it is also wise to understand their limits. Understanding the symptoms that necessitate medical attention is vital to ensuring safety and efficacy in self-care. For instance, deep cuts, severe burns, or persistent pain may require professional evaluation and treatment. Similarly, consulting a healthcare provider is essential if a condition does not improve with herbal treatment or worsens over time. This discernment ensures that herbal remedies complement conventional medicine, supporting overall health without compromising safety.

By integrating herbal first aid into your life, you embrace a tradition of natural healing that is both empowering and practical. These remedies provide a gentle, effective means of addressing common ailments, fostering a deeper connection with the healing power of nature. As you build your herbal first aid kit, you cultivate a sense of preparedness and confidence, ready to face the unexpected with grace and resilience.

Building a Home Apothecary: Essentials and Storage Tips

The idea of a home apothecary conjures images of jars filled with dried leaves and labeled bottles, each one a testament to the healing potential of nature's bounty. Creating your own space dedicated to herbal remedies is not just about collecting herbs; it's about creating a sanctuary to connect with the natural world and its healing gifts. To start building this personal haven, focus on selecting essential herbs that cater to your specific health needs. For many, this includes a selection of dried herbs for teas and tinctures, such as chamomile for relaxation, peppermint for digestion, and elderberry for immune support. These herbs serve as the foundation of your apothecary, ready to be transformed into soothing infusions or potent extracts.

Equally important are the tools and containers that house these botanical treasures. Airtight, dark containers are crucial for preserving the potency and safety of your herbal supplies. Opt for amber glass jars or metal tins, which offer optimal protection against environmental factors. Label each container with the herb's name, purchase date, and origin to help you track freshness and maintain an organized system. This straightforward practice ensures you know exactly what you have in stock and when you last replenished it, helping to prevent waste and extend the longevity of your inventory.

Proper storage is essential. Store your apothecary collection away from sunlight. Organizing your herbs by the expiry date, with the oldest at the front, helps you use them promptly and avoid spoilage. Regularly checking your supplies for signs of deterioration, such as discoloration or loss of aroma, ensures that you use only the freshest, most potent herbs in your preparations.

Maintaining a tidy and efficient apothecary space is essential for easy access to herbal remedies. Develop a labeling and categorization system that works for you, perhaps by grouping herbs according to their function—such as calming herbs, digestive aids, or immune boosters. This method lets you quickly locate the right herb for any situation, streamlining your preparation process. Consider using transparent labels for a clean, uniform look, and include relevant information like the herb's common and botanical names, along with any specific uses or precautions.

Personalizing your apothecary can be rewarding, allowing you to infuse your personality and creativity into the space. Consider Do It Yourself Projects (DIY) that enhance your herbal haven's function and beauty. For example, crafting custom herbal labels and storage jars can transform a simple shelf of bottles into a visually captivating display. Use decorative paper or fabric to craft unique labels, and experiment with various fonts and colors to express your style. Also, consider making storage containers, such as repurposed vintage jars or hand-painted tins, adding a touch of whimsy and charm to your collection.

These enhancements make your apothecary more inviting and deepen your connection to the herbs, turning each interaction into a mindful ritual. As you curate and care for your home apothecary, you cultivate a space that nurtures both body and spirit, a testament to the timeless wisdom of herbal medicine.

Herbal Self-Care Rituals: Nourishing Mind, Body, and Spirit

Imagine ending a long day with an inviting herbal bath, the warm water enveloping you in a cocoon of relaxation. Lavender and chamomile blossoms float gently around you, their soothing aromas mingling with the steam to ease tension in your body and mind. This experience is more than a bath; it is an intentional act of self-care that nourishes both body and spirit. Incorporating herbs into daily rituals like this can transform routine activities into powerful moments of healing and reflection. As you sink deeper into the water, you allow the stress of the day to dissolve, welcoming a sense of peace and rejuvenation.

Morning rituals can also benefit from the gentle power of herbs. Consider starting your day with meditation, accompanied by the calming scent of herbal incense. Sage, lemon balm, and other herbs can enhance your focus, grounding you for the day ahead. Lighting incense serves as a signal to your mind, inviting it to shift from the hurried thoughts of daily life to a place of quiet contemplation. Doing this cultivates mindfulness, encouraging you to carry calm and clarity into all your activities.

The intention behind these rituals amplifies their benefits. When you engage in herbal self-care with a clear purpose, you deepen the impact of each practice. Setting intentions for herbal use is a deliberate process that aligns your actions with your wellness goals. Before preparing your herbal bath, take a moment to reflect on what you hope to achieve—whether it's relaxation, healing, or mindfulness.

Integrating herbal practices with other self-care activities can create a holistic routine that addresses physical and emotional needs. For instance, a gentle herbal face steam offers a dual benefit of skincare and relaxation. As the steam opens your pores, allowing the beneficial compounds of herbs like calendula and rose to penetrate, you also enjoy the calming effect of the warm, aromatic mist. Similarly, an infused foot soak can relieve stress, soothing tired feet while encouraging overall relaxation. Adding herbs such as peppermint or eucalyptus to the water invigorates the senses, leaving you refreshed and revitalized.

Encouraging personalization and creativity in herbal rituals can enhance their effectiveness and enjoyment. We are unique, and our self-care practices should reflect that individuality. Keep a journal to document your herbal experiences and the effects you observe. This practice tracks your progress and is a reflective tool, helping you refine your rituals over time.

Herbal self-care rituals offer a meaningful way to connect with nature's healing gifts, nurturing every aspect of your being. By embracing these practices, you create a sanctuary of wellness within your daily life, a space where you can retreat and recharge. Let your creativity guide you as you explore the endless possibilities of herbal rituals, crafting a routine that is uniquely yours.

As we wrap up our exploration of how to seamlessly incorporate herbal remedies into your daily routine, it's clear that nature provides abundant tools for holistic well-being. Integrating plant-based medicine can be effortless and transformative, from morning teas and tinctures to herbal meals and self-care rituals. The key to success lies in consistency —when herbs become a natural part of your lifestyle, their benefits unfold gradually, creating lasting improvements in health and vitality.

As we embrace these practices, we must recognize that herbal medicine spans multiple cultures and traditions. Across the globe, diverse civilizations have long relied on the healing power of plants, each with its unique approaches and wisdom. Understanding these traditions deepens our appreciation for herbal medicine and broadens our perspective on using herbs effectively.

Herbal Remedies Across Cultures

Herbal healing is a universal language spoken by cultures across continents and generations. From the intricate formulas of Traditional Chinese Medicine (TCM) to the balancing principles of Ayurveda, the vibrant plant-based traditions of Africa, and the sacred remedies of Indigenous healers, every civilization has uniquely harnessed the power of herbs.

In Chapter 6, we'll journey through these global herbal traditions, uncovering how different cultures have cultivated, prepared, and utilized medicinal plants for healing and wellness. By exploring these time-honored practices, you'll understand how herbs have shaped human health for centuries and how these traditions can inspire your herbal journey.

Let's step into the world of herbal wisdom from across the globe.🌿✨

Herbal Remedies Across Cultures

"Ayurveda is a philosophy emphasizing balance, harmony, and the interconnectedness."

Picture yourself in a vibrant Indian marketplace, where the air is alive with the colors and aromas of spices and herbs. Vendors proudly display their turmeric, ginger, and ashwagandha, each claiming their products' unmatched quality. More than a healing method, Ayurveda is a philosophy emphasizing balance, harmony, and the interconnectedness of body, mind, and spirit, offering a rich heritage to those who embrace it.

Ayurvedic Herbal Practices: Aligning Doshas with Nature

Ayurvedic practices promote health and prevent disease through natural means, including diet, herbal remedies, lifestyle practices, and therapies. It aims to harmonize the body's energies.

The forces governing the physiological and psychological functions in the body are the three doshas: Pitta, Vata, and Kapha. Each person has a unique balance of these powers, which influence them physically and mentally.

These doshas—Vata, Pitta, and Kapha—represent different elements of nature and influence our physical and mental characteristics. Vata, linked to the elements of air and space, controls movement and is marked by qualities of lightness and coolness. Those with a dominant Vata may experience restlessness and anxiety when out of balance. Pitta, linked to fire and water, regulates metabolism and digestion, often manifesting as heat and intensity. An imbalanced Pitta can lead to irritability and inflammation. Kapha, embodying Earth and water, provides structure and stability, but an excess can cause lethargy and congestion. The delicate dance of these doshas determines our overall health and well-being.

Herbs are the unsung heroes in the Ayurvedic quest for balance. They play a pivotal role in restoring equilibrium to the doshas, offering tailored remedies for each individual's needs. Ashwagandha, a revered adaptogen, is particularly beneficial for stabilizing Vata. Its warming properties counteract Vata's coolness, grounding the mind and body. This herb often alleviates stress and promotes restful sleep, helping those with Vata imbalances find calm and stability. Triphala, a potent blend of three fruits—Amla (Indian gooseberry), Haritaki, and Bibhitaki—plays a significant role in traditional Ayurvedic cleansing practices. This herbal blend supports digestion and strengthens resilience, demonstrating the individualized nature of Ayurvedic remedies.

Herbal decoctions, known as "kashayas," are a standard preparation method. These involve boiling herbs in water to extract their essence, creating a concentrated liquid that we can consume for its therapeutic benefits. Pastes, or "lepas," are another traditional preparation, often applied topically to treat skin conditions and inflammation. The use of ghee, a clarified butter, as a carrier substance is also prevalent in Ayurveda. Ghee enhances the absorption of herbs, acting as a vehicle to deliver their healing properties deep into the tissues. This method maximizes efficacy and nourishes the body at a cellular level.

By embracing the principles of Ayurveda, individuals like Ravi (those who integrate Ayurvedic principles and practices into their lives) can cultivate a deeper connection with their bodies and the natural world.

Ayurveda promotes holistic wellness, including physical, mental, and spiritual well-being. This comprehensive system encourages individuals to align their lifestyle with their unique constitution, fostering a balanced and healthy life.

Exercise: Discovering Your Dosha

To further explore the world of Ayurveda, take a moment to identify your dominant dosha. Reflect on your physical and emotional characteristics, considering elements like body type, energy levels, and temperament. Use these insights to guide your choice of herbs and lifestyle practices, aligning your daily routine with your unique constitution supporting your holistic well-being.

Ayurveda invites you to see yourself as part of a larger tapestry, interconnected with nature and its rhythms.

By understanding and balancing your doshas, you can tap into the potential of herbal remedies to improve your health and vitality. This ancient wisdom provides a timeless and personal approach to wellness, empowering you to make informed choices that enhance your holistic well-being. It encourages you to embrace the healing power of nature on your journey toward holistic health, giving you the control and proactivity to shape your well-being.

Traditional Chinese Medicine: Balancing Yin and Yang with Herbs

Within Chinese traditional medicine lies the profound concept of Yin and Yang, two complementary forces reflecting a state of equilibrium and peaceful coexistence with the larger cosmic order and, by extension, within the human body. Yin embodies coolness, rest, and introspection, while Yang signifies warmth, activity, and extroversion. According to TCM, health is a dynamic equilibrium between these forces; illness arises when one dominates or is deficient. Qi, the vital life force that flows through the body, is the medium through which Yin and Yang manifest. This life force circulates through meridians, akin to energy highways, and any obstruction or imbalance that leads to physical and mental challenges. Herbs play a crucial role in facilitating this balance, acting as agents to restore harmony and promote the smooth flow of Qi.

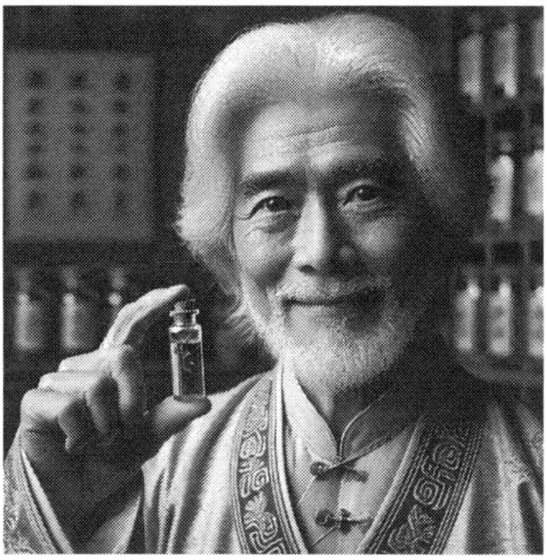

Here is a new artistic representation of the Yin and Yang concept in Traditional Chinese Medicine. It visually expresses the balance between Yin (coolness, rest, introspection) and Yang (warmth, activity, energy) while incorporating a flowing Qi energy stream that weaves through the Yin-Yang symbol, symbolizing the life force circulating through the body.

Key herbs in TCM serve distinct functions based on their properties and the balance they aim to restore. For instance, ginseng is considered a master herb renowned for enhancing Qi. Ginseng's ability to help the body adapt to stress and maintain balance, bolstering energy levels and mental clarity, is well known. By invigorating Qi, Ginseng supports the body's resilience and vitality, making it invaluable for those experiencing depletion or weakness. Reishi mushroom, another staple of TCM, is celebrated for its immune-supporting properties, helping to modulate the immune system, enhance sleep, and reduce stress, aligning with the TCM principle of maintaining balance and preventing disease. These herbs exemplify how TCM employs natural remedies to address imbalances, restoring the body's innate harmony and giving hope for a healthier future.

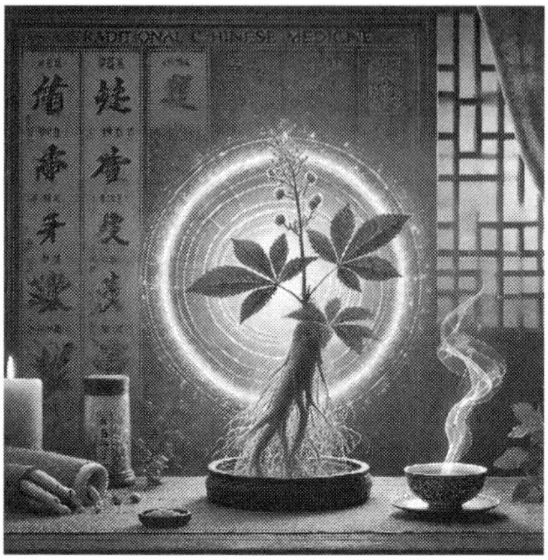

Here is your image depicting a serene traditional Chinese medicine scene featuring a radiant ginseng plant glowing with golden energy, symbolizing its power to enhance Qi. The background includes a tranquil herbalist's study, ancient scrolls, and a steaming cup of ginseng tea, evoking balance, harmony, and rejuvenation.

The preparation of herbal remedies in TCM is an art refined over centuries. Herbal teas, or "tisanes," are a typical preparation involving steeping herbs in hot water to extract their healing properties. This method is particularly effective for herbs that release their active compounds into water, providing a gentle yet potent remedy. Infused with medicinal herbs, Soups offer another means of delivering therapeutic benefits. These soups are nutritious and serve as a vehicle for herbs that work best when consumed with food, enhancing digestion and assimilation. Acupuncture often complements herbal treatment, targeting specific meridians to facilitate the movement of Qi and improve the efficacy of herbal remedies. This integrative approach underscores the holistic nature of TCM, where herbs, diet, and physical therapies work in concert to promote health.

Traditional Chinese Medicine (TCM) plays a significant role in shaping and reflecting the culture and history of Chinese civilization. The development and practices of TCM are closely linked with the evolution of Chinese society, influencing and being influenced by its cultural and historical context. TCM and Chinese civilization have grown and evolved together, enriching and informing the other.

From ancient dynasties to the present, herbal medicine has been the center of health practices in China. Ancient texts like the Shennong Bencaojing chronicle the use of hundreds of medicinal herbs, showcasing a deep reservoir of botanical wisdom refined over thousands of years. These records serve as a testament to the enduring legacy of herbal medicine, preserving invaluable knowledge passed down through generations. Within imperial courts, herbalists were held in the highest regard, entrusted with safeguarding the health and longevity of emperors and their families. Their mastery of medicinal plants and healing formulations was a closely guarded tradition.

Understanding and using herbs are deeply ingrained within the Chinese culture and have been passed down over thousands of years. Chinese herbal medicine is celebrated with seasonal festivals and has a global reach and influence. The key concepts like Qi (a vital life force flowing through all living things that maintains balance and harmony in the body and mind), Yin (willpower and intention that drives focused thoughts and purposeful actions, and inward movement), and Yang (active, warm, and energetic qualities, embodying brightness and outward movement), and the use of herbs are known by many who want a balanced life. These principles help us understand the connection between the environment, body, and mind.

This reverence for herbal wisdom extends beyond the royal palaces into the daily lives of the Chinese people. The seasonal festivals and rituals incorporate her people and the natural world, a practical and spiritual connection.

Indigenous Herbal Wisdom: Lessons from Native Traditions

Picture a vast expanse of wild prairie, where the wind gently moves, carrying the tales and histories of those ancient peoples who have walked these lands for millennia. For indigenous cultures, plants are more than just physical remedies; they embody the spirit and energy of the Earth, forming an integral part of their healing practices. These communities view plants as sentient beings, each with a unique essence and purpose. This perspective fosters a profound respect for nature and its gifts, where herbs are not merely tools for healing but partners in the journey toward well-being. In many indigenous traditions, the spirit of a plant is invoked during healing ceremonies, enhancing the plant's efficacy.

Herbs are deeply interwoven into indigenous communities' spiritual and cultural traditions, serving as sacred tools in ceremonies that honor the interconnectedness of all life. People particularly revere sage for its purifying properties. People traditionally burn it in smudging rituals, believing its fragrant smoke cleanses individuals, spaces, and objects, dispelling negative energy and restoring balance and harmony.

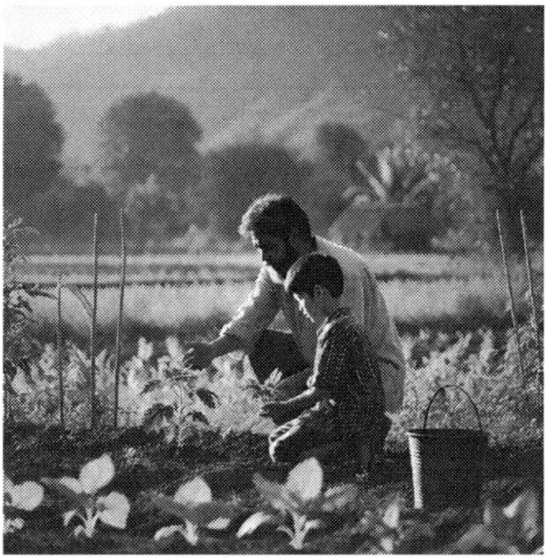

The image depicts Indigenous Herbal Wisdom, showcasing the sacred connection between nature, plants, and healing traditions.

This practice transcends symbolism; it is a ritual that reinforces one's connection to the natural world and the ancestors who came before. Another vital herb is sweetgrass, which promotes peace and harmony with its sweet, vanilla-like scent. When braided and burned in ceremonies, sweetgrass is said to invite positive energy and create a sense of balance and tranquility. These herbs act as bridges between the physical and spiritual realms, with their use deeply rooted in tradition and significance.

The transmission of herbal knowledge within Indigenous communities exemplifies the power of oral traditions and storytelling. Elders are often viewed as keepers of this wisdom, passing down their knowledge through narratives rich in cultural context and ancestral memory. These stories are more than just instructional; they represent living histories that embody the community's values, beliefs, and practices.

Through storytelling, young generations learn the significance of each plant, its properties, and the rituals associated with its use. This method of teaching ensures that herbal wisdom is not only preserved but also adapted to the changing needs of the community. It fosters a sense of identity and continuity, linking past, present, and future in a seamless flow of knowledge.

Examples of successful indigenous herbal practices abound, illustrating the profound impact of these traditions on health and wellness. Community healing circles, where individuals gather to share and receive healing, are a cornerstone of indigenous health practices. In these circles, herbal remedies are often combined with prayer, song, and other spiritual elements to create a holistic healing experience. For instance, in some Native American communities, individuals may use a mixture of sage and cedar in a steam bath to promote respiratory health and spiritual cleansing. Participants emerge physically rejuvenated and spiritually uplifted, strengthening their sense of connectedness to the community and the Earth.

In another example, herbal poultices and teas typically address colds, digestive issues, and skin conditions. These remedies are crafted with care, using locally sourced plants gathered with respect for the natural environment. Sacred rituals often enrich the preparation of these herbal remedies, honoring the spirit of the plants and the healing intentions behind their use.

These ceremonial practices reflect the deeply holistic approach of indigenous healing traditions, where physical, emotional, and spiritual well-being are seamlessly interconnected. This interconnection reinforces the belief that true healing extends beyond the body to encompass the mind and soul.

This approach to health emphasizes balance and harmony, principles that resonate deeply with those who seek a more integrated path to wellness.

Their knowledge offers valuable insights into sustainable living and the respectful use of natural resources. As you explore these traditions, consider the lessons they impart—lessons of reverence for nature, the power of community, and the enduring wisdom of the Earth. These teachings remind us that healing is not just about treating symptoms but about fostering a deep relationship with the world around us. In doing so, we honor the legacy of those who have come before us and carry their wisdom into the future.

European Herbal Medicine: The Roots of Modern Practices

In the quiet corridors of medieval monasteries, a tradition of herbal medicine quietly flourished, sowing the seeds for what would become a cornerstone of European health practices. Monastic herbalists, often monks dedicated to studying nature and healing, meticulously cultivated gardens brimming with medicinal plants. These monks compiled their knowledge into herbals—detailed manuscripts describing plants' uses and properties. Individuals preserved and expanded the healing arts in these sacred spaces, bridging ancient Roman and Greek practices into the Middle Ages. As Europe moved into the Renaissance, this era of rebirth saw herbalism reach new heights. With increased access to classical texts and a burgeoning interest in science and nature, herbalists began looking at plants with renewed vigor. The Renaissance brought forth figures like Nicholas Culpeper, whose seminal work, "The Complete Herbal," democratized herbal knowledge and made it accessible to the broader public. His writings combined personal observations with traditional lore, creating a rich tapestry of herbal wisdom that continues to influence herbalists today.

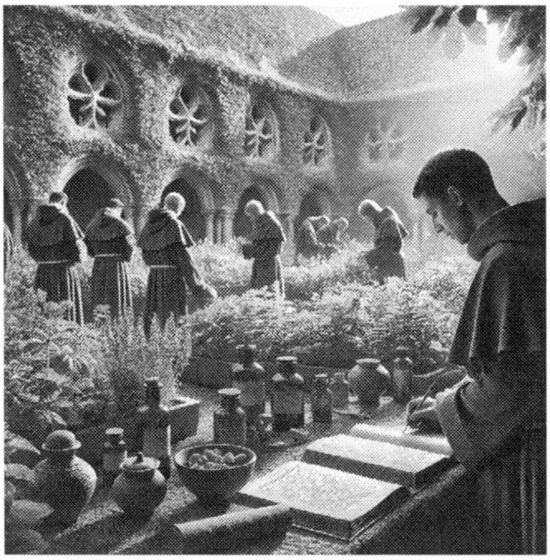

Here is the recreated image of a medieval monastery garden with monks in traditional robes tending to medicinal plants, documenting herbal knowledge, and preparing remedies. Throughout this rich history, certain herbs have endured, becoming staples in European herbal medicine.

St. John's Wort, recognized for its bright yellow flowers, has long been valued for its mood-enhancing qualities. Traditionally used to ward off melancholy and boost mental well-being, it remains a popular choice for those seeking natural remedies for mild depression and anxiety. Yarrow, another enduring favorite, was historically prized for its ability to staunch wounds and prevent infection. Roman soldiers famously carried it into battle, using it to treat injuries on the field. Its astringent qualities and ability to promote healing made yarrow an indispensable component of the herbalist's toolkit.

Here is the realistic close-up of a St. John's Wort (Hypericum perforatum) plant in full bloom, featuring its bright yellow flowers with delicate petals and characteristic tiny black dots.

European folklore and culture have also played a significant role in shaping the use of herbs. Herbal remedies often appear in fairy tales and myths passed down through generations of storytellers, imbuing them with magical properties and symbolic meanings. These stories not only served as entertainment but also as a means of preserving and transmitting knowledge about the healing powers of plants. The tale of Rapunzel, for instance, intertwines the use of rampion—a leafy plant believed to possess restorative properties—with themes of desire and healing. Such narratives embedded herbal knowledge within the cultural fabric, ensuring its survival despite scientific skepticism and societal change.

Today, the legacy of European herbal medicine is alive and well, and you may find them in modern practices like naturopathy and homeopathy. These disciplines integrate traditional European herbal wisdom with contemporary scientific understanding, offering holistic approaches to health and wellness. Naturopathy, which emphasizes the body's intrinsic ability to heal, often incorporates European herbs such as nettle and chamomile for their detoxifying and calming effects. Homeopathy, with its principle of "like cures like," utilizes highly diluted substances, including herbs, to stimulate the body's healing response. Both fields exemplify the enduring impact of European herbal traditions, adapting age-old practices to meet the needs of today's health-conscious individuals.

In essence, the evolution of European herbal medicine reflects a continuous dialogue between past and present, where ancient practices inform modern applications. The monastic gardens and Renaissance herbals laid the foundational knowledge that empowers contemporary practitioners to explore the vast potential of plants. By embracing these traditions, we gain valuable health tools and a deeper appreciation for the wisdom of the natural world. The stories and practices of European herbal medicine remind us that healing is a dynamic, living process—a dance between history and innovation, culture and science.

African Herbal Traditions: Understanding the Legacy of Healing

Picture the vast landscapes of Africa, from the sprawling savannas to the dense rainforests (for example, the Congo Basin, the world's second-largest rainforest after the Amazon), each teeming with a diversity of plant life that has shaped the continent's rich herbal traditions.

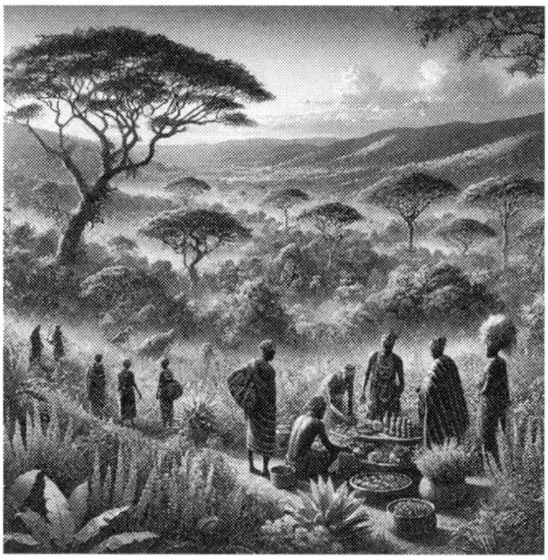

The image represents African Herbal Traditions, showcasing traditional healers and herbalists in a vibrant natural setting, deeply connected to the land and its botanical wisdom.

Across Africa, herbal practices are as varied as the ecosystems, reflecting each region's unique flora and fauna. Traditional healers and herbalists, often revered within their communities, hold the keys to this botanical wisdom. They draw upon a profound understanding of the local environment and its medicinal plants to treat ailments and promote health. This knowledge passed down through generations, is integral to cultural identity and survival, rooted in the belief that nature provides a remedy for every ailment.

Among the many herbs cherished in African traditional medicine, neem stands out for its remarkable antibacterial properties. Known as the "village pharmacy," neem's leaves, bark, and oil combat infections and support skin health. It is a staple in many households, used in remedies that range from toothpaste to insect repellent. Its versatility and effectiveness have made it a cornerstone of herbal medicine in African regions. Rooibos, another significant herb, is renowned for its antioxidant benefits. Indigenous to South Africa's Cederberg Mountains, rooibos is a caffeine-free tea celebrated for its soothing properties and supporting heart and skin health.

People worldwide have noted its rich red hue and unique flavor, yet its roots remain deeply embedded in African tradition. African herbalism greatly emphasizes the spiritual significance of herbs. Plants are not merely physical entities but imbued with spiritual energy and importance. They play a vital role in rituals and ceremonies designed to heal the body and the spirit. Herbs such as African wormwood and buchu, often used in rituals, aim to purify spaces and individuals by removing or neutralizing negative energies. Practitioners intend these purification rituals to create a more harmonious and positive environment.

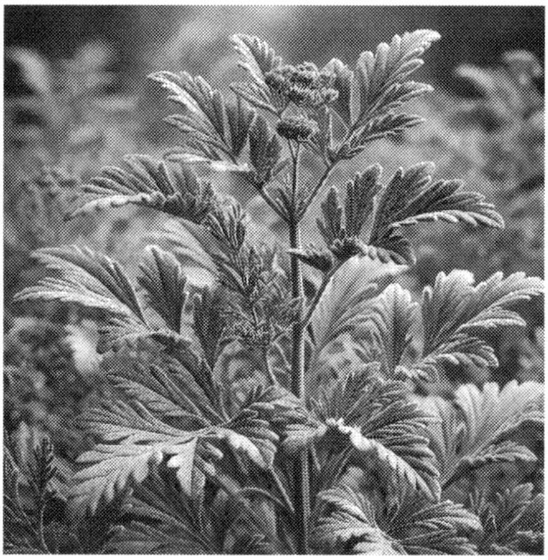

Here is the image of an African Wormwood (Artemisia afra) plant, showcasing its silvery-green feathery leaves and tiny yellow flower buds in a natural setting with soft sunlight.

This spiritual dimension of herbalism underscores the holistic approach to health that characterizes many African traditions, where the physical, emotional, and spiritual are interconnected. People view healing as a communal and sacred act, often involving music, dance, and prayer to enhance the efficacy of the herbs and the overall experience.

Efforts to preserve and revive African herbal knowledge are gaining momentum, recognizing the risk of losing this invaluable cultural heritage in the face of modernization and globalization. Initiatives to document traditional herbal practices are underway. These efforts seek to catalog the extensive knowledge of plants and their uses, ensuring it is accessible to future generations.

The legacy of African herbalism is a testament to nature's enduring power and the human spirit's resilience. It offers a rich tapestry of healing that transcends time and borders.

SOUTH AMERICAN PLANTS: AMAZONIAN HERBAL REMEDIES

The Amazon rainforest is a vast expanse teeming with life. It is home to countless species that exist nowhere else on the planet. This lush, vibrant ecosystem, spanning several countries in South America, is a treasure trove of biodiversity. The rainforest's dense canopy shelters many plants, and modern science has yet to discover many of them. With their unique chemical compositions, these plants have been used for centuries by indigenous tribes for their healing properties. We cannot overstate the ecological significance of the Amazon; it serves as a reservoir of genetic diversity and a vital component of the global climate system.

Within this rich tapestry of plant life lies a world of medicinal herbs, each with its own story and use. Among these, Ayahuasca stands out for its profound spiritual significance. This potent brew, made from the Banisteriopsis caapi vine and other Amazonian plants, is used in traditional healing ceremonies to foster spiritual insight and personal transformation. The effects of Ayahuasca are both powerful and introspective, often leading participants to explore the deepest recesses of their consciousness. It is not merely a medicine but a gateway to understanding one's place in the universe and the interconnectedness of all life.

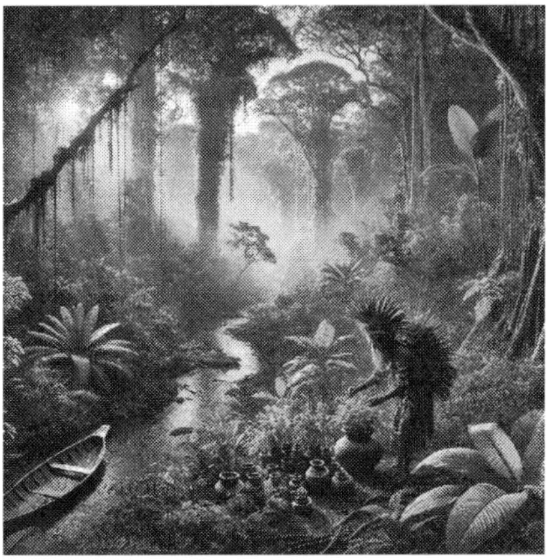

The scene represents Amazonian Herbal Remedies, featuring the lush Amazon rainforest, an indigenous healer selecting medicinal plants, and a canoe by the riverbank.

Indigenous peoples have utilized the remarkable Cat's Claw, a climbing vine with unique claw-shaped thorns, to address ailments ranging from arthritis to digestive issues. The active compounds in Cat's Claw (alkaloids and flavonoids) interact to boost our body's ability to defend itself against illnesses. As a result, it has gained popularity in the global wellness market, where its benefits are increasingly recognized by those seeking natural alternatives to conventional treatments.

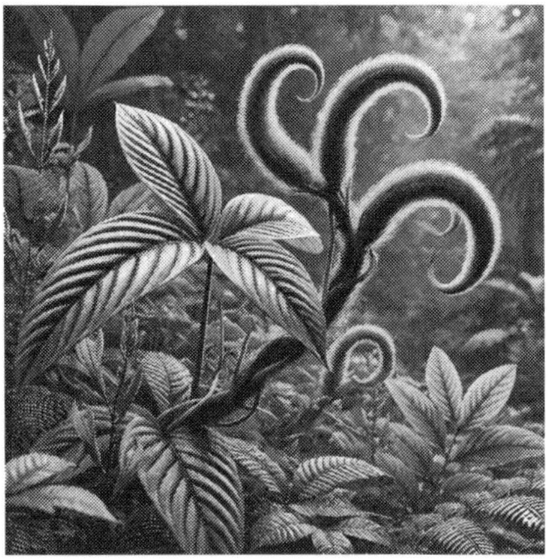

Here is a realistic close-up of a Cat's Claw plant (Uncaria tomentosa) growing in its natural rainforest habitat. The plant features vibrant green leaves with distinctive curved claw-like structures on its vines and small yellowish flowers.

The indigenous knowledge systems that have preserved the use of these plants are as intricate and diverse as the rainforest itself. Amazonian tribes revere shamans and healers as custodians of this ancestral wisdom. They deeply intertwine their understanding of plant medicine with spiritual practices, where the physical and metaphysical realms converge.

Shamans often undergo rigorous training, learning to communicate with the plants' spirit and harness their healing powers. This sacred knowledge is protected and passed down through generations, ensuring its continuity and adaptation to changing times.

Integrating Amazonian herbs into contemporary wellness practices is becoming more prevalent in modern contexts. The adaptogenic properties of certain plants, such as Maca and Guayusa, are being harnessed in global markets to support energy and resilience. These herbs, celebrated for their ability to help the body adapt to stress, are now featured in supplements, teas, and health foods worldwide. The increasing interest in Amazonian herbs reflects a growing recognition of their potential to enhance well-being in today's fast-paced world. This fusion of traditional knowledge and modern application offers a promising frontier for personal health and sustainable development.

The journey through the Amazon's herbal landscape reveals a profound connection between nature and healing, one that transcends cultural and geographical boundaries. The Amazon's wealth of medicinal plants provides solutions for contemporary health challenges and offers insights into the intricate web of life that sustains us all.

The wisdom we gain from Amazonian herbal traditions highlights the enduring knowledge of indigenous cultures and their crucial role in promoting a holistic approach to health and wellness.

Across the world, diverse cultures have long embraced the healing power of plants, each tradition adding a unique layer to the vast and evolving story of herbal medicine. From the ancient formulas of Traditional Chinese Medicine to the sacred plant rituals of indigenous communities, these traditions offer timeless wisdom that continues to inspire modern herbal practices. Understanding and honoring these cultural approaches enriches our wellness journeys and fosters a deeper appreciation for the interconnectedness of nature and human health.

As we move forward, we step beyond foundational herbal knowledge and into the realm of advanced herbal practices. The next chapter delves into powerful herbal techniques, from synergistic herb combinations to seasonal herbalism and fermentation methods. Whether you are looking to refine your skills or explore innovative ways to maximize the potency of plant medicine, Chapter 7 will guide you into the art and science of advanced herbal mastery.

For those ready to elevate their herbal journey, mastering advanced herbal practices unlocks a new level of potency and effectiveness. Herbal medicine is not just about individual plants; it's about how they work together, how they interact with our bodies, and how preparation methods can enhance their healing potential.

In this chapter, we will explore:

- 🌿 Herbal Synergy – How combining specific herbs amplifies their benefits
- 🍂 Seasonal Herbalism – Aligning plant remedies with nature's cycles
- 🧪 Fermented Herbal Remedies – Boosting bioavailability through fermentation
- 🌱 Wildcrafting with Care – Ethical foraging techniques for sustainability
- 🍷 Herbal Vinegars & Oxymels – Ancient methods with modern applications

By integrating these advanced techniques, you'll better understand how to craft and refine herbal preparations, ensuring maximum potency, sustainability, and alignment with your wellness goals. Get ready to dive deeper into the alchemy of herbal medicine and elevate your practice to new heights!🌿✨

Advanced Herbal Practices

"Unlock the secrets of herbal synergy to crystallize nature's healing power and enhance your well-being."

In my herb garden, I find solace and inspiration. The vibrant hues and rich scents of plants remind me of the profound synergy within the natural world. This synergy, a harmonious interplay between different elements, is a potent concept in herbal medicine. Herbal synergy is the combined effect of two or more herbs greater than the sum of their individual effects. When we combine certain herbs, their properties can merge, creating a blend more significant than the sum of its parts. This principle of herbal synergy is both an art and a science, offering us the potential to craft more potent and effective remedies.

Understanding the potent concept of herbal synergy empowers us and gives us the control to craft remedies that align with our unique needs. This knowledge instills deep confidence in our herbal practices, as we know we can create remedies that work for us.

A key advantage is the undeniable power of herbal synergy in bolstering the immune system. By thoughtfully combining herbs that complement each other, we can significantly enhance their collective ability to fortify our body's defenses. This comprehensive defense strategy ensures you feel secure and protected, boosting your confidence in your health.

Stress relief is another area where herbal synergy shines, particularly when integrating nervines and adaptogens. Nervines like passionflower and adaptogens such as ashwagandha can work together to soothe the nervous system and enhance resilience to stress. Passionflower calms the mind by influencing neurotransmitter activity, while ashwagandha helps regulate or adjust the body's cortisol amount. Combining these herbs creates a balanced formulation that addresses immediate stress and long-term resilience, offering holistic support for the mind and body.

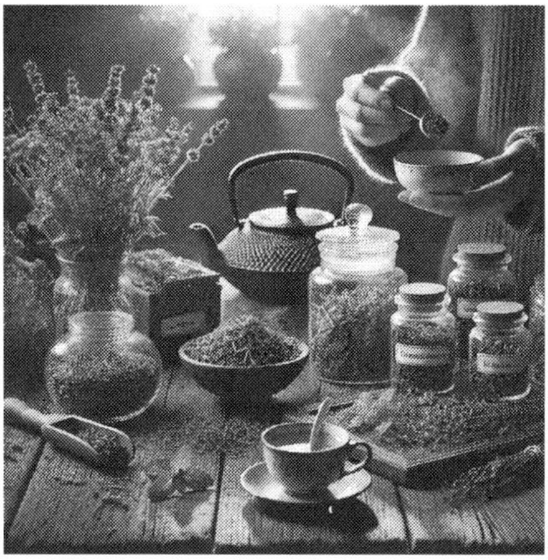

Creating effective herbal combinations is an art that requires a nuanced understanding of each herb's properties and how they interact. It's crucial to balance contrasting qualities to avoid diminishing their effects. For example, pairing a warming herb like ginger with a cooling one like peppermint can create a balanced digestive tonic. Ginger stimulates digestion and enhances circulation, while peppermint soothes and relaxes the digestive tract. When understood and applied correctly, this complementary pairing harnesses the strengths of both herbs, providing comprehensive support for digestive health and showcasing your knowledge and skill in herbal practices.

Avoiding antagonistic combinations that could counteract each other's benefits is crucial when blending herbs. For instance, combining a potent stimulant like ginseng with a sedative like valerian may lead to conflicting outcomes, diminishing the effectiveness of both. Similarly, mixing herbs with different effects on blood pressure or blood sugar levels can be counterproductive. Understanding these interactions ensures that the synergy of your blends is positive and beneficial.

Ginger and turmeric are among the most popular and effective herbal combinations for overall wellness. Both herbs possess potent anti-inflammatory properties, making them powerful allies in reducing inflammation and promoting joint health. Ginger's active compounds, gingerols and shogaols, work synergistically with turmeric's curcumin to enhance their anti-inflammatory effects. This combination relieves pain and inflammation and supports overall vitality and longevity.

Pairing peppermint with chamomile for digestive support creates a soothing blend that calms and nurtures the digestive system. Peppermint's menthol content relaxes the gastrointestinal tract, alleviating symptoms of indigestion and bloating. Chamomile, known for its gentle calming effects, reduces stress-related digestive issues. Together, they form a harmonious blend that supports digestive health and promotes relaxation.

When you add essential oils to your daily routine, you must ensure they are diluted correctly before applying them to your skin. Dilution helps prevent skin irritation or adverse reactions since essential oils are highly concentrated. Additionally, you should be cautious with phototoxic oils like bergamot and lemon. Proper dilution and awareness of phototoxic oils ensure successful use without harming your skin.

Individual tolerances vary; what works well for one person may not suit another. Monitoring for allergic reactions is crucial, especially when experimenting with new combinations. Start small. See how your body responds, then go from there. As you get more comfortable, you can increase the amount. This awareness of potential risks and precautions is essential for a safe and effective herbal practice, providing you with reassurance and safety.

Touching base with your doctor is always a smart thing to do, mainly if you take medications or have underlying health conditions. Some herbs can interact with pharmaceuticals, altering their effects or leading to adverse reactions. By seeking professional guidance, you can ensure that your herbal practices are safe and effective, complementing your overall health regimen and providing you with reassurance and safety.

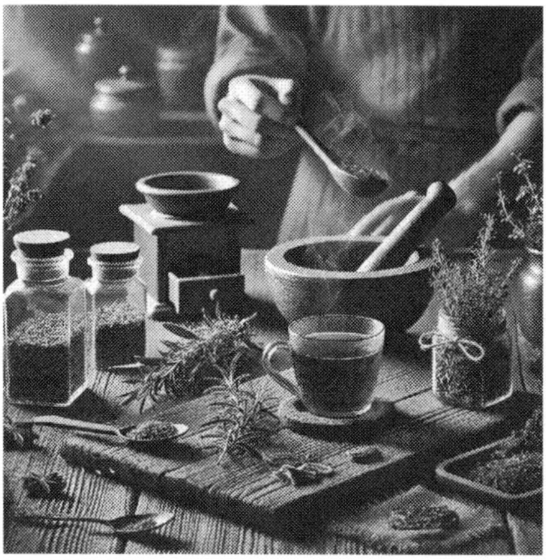

INTERACTIVE ELEMENT: CREATE YOUR SYNERGISTIC BLEND

Interactive Element: Create Your Synergistic Blend. Select two or three herbs that resonate with your wellness goals. Consider their individual properties and how they might complement each other. For instance, if you want to boost your immune system, choose echinacea for its immune-stimulating properties and elderberry for its antiviral effects. Create a small batch of your blend, noting the proportions and your rationale for selecting each herb. Record your observations and any effects you notice as you use your blend. This exercise enhances your understanding of herbal synergy and empowers you to craft personalized remedies that align with your unique needs.

SEASONAL HERBALISM: ADAPTING PRACTICES THROUGHOUT THE YEAR

The changing seasons bring a rhythm to our lives, influencing not only the environment around us but also our internal balance. Seasonal herbalism embraces this natural cycle, adapting practices to align with each season's unique needs and energies. This approach enhances the effectiveness of herbal remedies. In the depths of winter, when the cold seeps into our bones, warming herbs like ginger and cinnamon provide comfort and vitality. These herbs generate internal heat, improving circulation and bolstering the immune system to ward off winter ailments. With its spicy warmth, ginger tea becomes a daily ritual, infusing our bodies with energy and resilience.

Each season invites us to embrace specific herbal strategies that cater to its distinct characteristics. Spring, with its promise of renewal, is the ideal time for detoxification. Dandelion, cherished for its cleansing properties, supports liver function and aids in flushing out accumulated toxins. A simple dandelion root tea, earthy and grounding, helps clear the system, preparing us for the vibrant energy of the warmer months. As summer fades into fall, we focus on fortifying our defenses against the coming cold. Elderberry, renowned for its antiviral properties, has become a staple. Its rich, dark berries are transformed into soothing syrups and immune-boosting teas, bolstering our natural defenses and protecting us from seasonal illnesses. These practices support physical health and create rituals that ground us in the present moment, fostering mindfulness and gratitude.

Seasonal transitions can be challenging as our bodies adjust to new temperatures and rhythms. Herbal formulations tailored to these transitions offer support and ease discomfort. A seasonal tea blend, carefully crafted to balance energy and mood, can help harmonize these shifts. For instance, a chamomile, lavender, and lemon balm blend calms the nervous system, alleviating the stress of change and promoting restful sleep. Similarly, herbal baths infused with rosemary and eucalyptus rejuvenate and refresh, helping shake off the previous season's remnants and embrace the new. These formulations provide physical benefits and a sense of ritual and continuity, connecting us to the cycles of nature.

Worldwide cultural practices have long recognized the importance of aligning herbal practices with the seasons. "Seasonal herbs closely tie to cultural activities in China. For example, during the Dragon Boat Festival, aromatic herbs like mugwort and calamus are hung in homes to ward off disease, reflecting an understanding of these plants' protective qualities.

Similarly, in many Indigenous cultures, seasonal gatherings and ceremonies incorporate specific herbs that align with the energies of that time, honoring the interconnectedness of people, plants, and the earth. These practices remind us of the wisdom embedded in our ancestral traditions, offering guidance and inspiration for our modern herbal journeys.

Fermentation in Herbal Medicine: Kombucha, Kefir, and More

In herbal medicine, fermentation is a transformative process that enhances herbs' nutritional and medicinal properties. It's a time-honored tradition that not only preserves the integrity of these plants but also unlocks beneficial compounds, making them more accessible to our bodies. Fermentation introduces probiotics—live bacteria and yeasts beneficial for gut health—into herbal preparations, thus creating a symbiotic relationship between herbs and microbes. These probiotics aid digestion, boost the immune system, and improve overall well-being.

Fermentation helps preserve herbal products, making them last longer without spoiling. Additionally, fermentation maintains the strength and effectiveness of the herbs' beneficial properties. This dual effect makes fermentation a valuable method for extending the shelf life of herbal preparations while keeping them potent and effective.

This dual benefit of enhanced nutrition and preservation makes fermentation a valuable technique in the herbalist's toolkit.

Among the array of fermented herbal products, kombucha and kefir are particularly popular. Kombucha, a fizzy, tangy tea, is often infused with herbs like ginger and lemon balm to enhance its health benefits and flavor profile. With its anti-inflammatory properties, ginger complements the digestive benefits of kombucha, while lemon balm adds a calming, citrusy note, perfect for stress relief. Kefir, another fermented beverage, can be infused with chamomile to create a soothing drink that promotes relaxation and digestive wellness. Chamomile's gentle, calming effects blend seamlessly with kefir's probiotic benefits, offering a multifaceted approach to health.

Crafting fermented herbal products at home can be a fulfilling experience. You can explore new flavors and customize blends to suit your health requirements. To prepare an herbal kombucha starter, begin with a batch of sweetened tea. Once cooled, add a SCOBY—a symbiotic culture of bacteria and yeast—and some starter liquid from a previous batch.

After this initial fermentation, you can introduce your chosen herbs. Add slices of fresh ginger and sprigs of lemon balm, seal the jar, and allow it to ferment for a few more days until it develops a balanced taste.

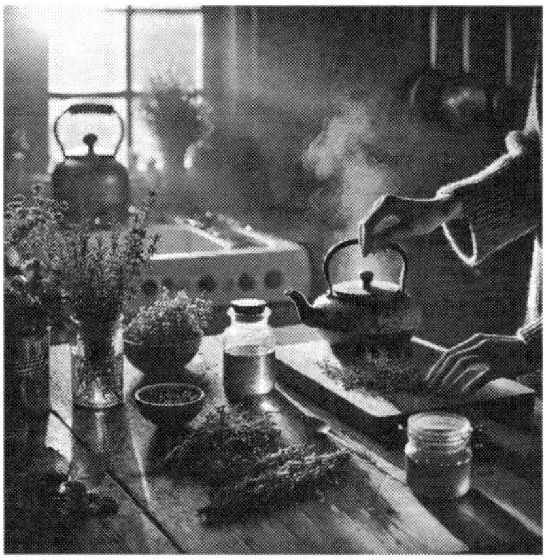

For kefir, start with kefir grains, clusters of beneficial bacteria and yeast. Combine these grains with milk (or a non-dairy alternative) in a jar, cover it with a breathable cloth, and leave it at room temperature for 24 to 48 hours. Once the kefir has thickened and tastes tangy, strain out the grains and infuse the liquid with chamomile flowers. Let this mixture sit for a few hours to allow the chamomile to impart its flavor and properties, then refrigerate.

Safety and storage are crucial components of successful fermentation. Constantly monitor your fermenting products for signs of mold or off smells indicating contamination. Mold, recognizable by its fuzzy appearance, should be discarded immediately to prevent health risks. Keep your equipment sterile and ensure that your fermentation environment is clean. Once your kombucha or kefir is ready, please keep it in a cool place like the refrigerator to slow further fermentation and maintain its flavor and potency. Proper storage preserves the quality of your fermented products and extends their shelf life, allowing you to enjoy them over time.

Fermented herbal beverages bridge the ancient wisdom of herbal medicine and modern nutritional science. They provide a dynamic way to incorporate the benefits of herbs and probiotics into your diet, enhancing your physical health and connection to herbalism traditions. As you explore the world of fermented herbs, you'll discover flavors and health benefits that enrich your herbal practice and life.

Wildcrafting: Advanced Techniques for Experienced Foragers

In the serene stillness of a forest, the air is thick with the scent of earth and greenery. A wealth of wild herbs is waiting to be found among the towering trees and whispering leaves.

For those who have honed their skills in wildcrafting, these natural landscapes offer a canvas rich with opportunity but also demand a deep respect and understanding of sustainable harvesting practices. As an advanced forager, you must identify rare and potent herbs—those hidden gems that require knowledge and keen observation.

Ghost pipe, a peculiar plant devoid of chlorophyll, stands out with its ghostly white appearance. Revered for its pain-relieving properties, it is a treasure for those who seek natural analgesics. However, its rarity necessitates a gentle touch, as overharvesting can threaten its delicate populations.

Navigating the diverse ecosystems where these herbs grow requires understanding the subtle nuances within each environment. Forests, fields, and wetlands each present their own unique set of challenges and rewards. Recognizing microclimates—small, distinct climate zones within a larger area—can significantly enhance your foraging success. The canopy creates a cooler, shaded microclimate in a dense forest, ideal for shade-loving plants like wild ginger. Conversely, open fields bask in sunlight, nurturing sun-loving herbs like yarrow. Wetlands, with their abundance of moisture, support plants like cattail and marshmallow, which are known for their soothing properties. By observing these microclimates, you can adapt your foraging strategies to suit the specific conditions of each terrain, maximizing the diversity and abundance of your harvest.

However, with the privilege of wildcrafting comes a profound responsibility. The ethical considerations of this practice are paramount, guiding every decision you make in the field. As caretakers or guardians of the land, we are responsible for ensuring that our activities do not harm or lead to the reduction of fragile or endangered plant species. It's a call to be mindful and conscientious about our environmental impact.

Always consult resources like the United Plant Savers to verify the conservation status of the plants you intend to harvest. Furthermore, promoting biodiversity through careful harvesting practices is crucial. Taking only the needed resources and rotating your foraging sites allows plant populations to thrive and regenerate, supporting the intricate web of life that depends on these ecosystems.

You may encounter nettles while exploring lesser-known wild herbs, a plant often overlooked due to its stinging reputation. Yet, when handled with care, nettles unveil their potential as a nutrient-rich powerhouse, abundant in vitamins and minerals. Once dried or cooked, their leaves lose their sting and become a valuable addition to teas and soups, significantly boosting your body's vitality. Another intriguing find is the ghost pipe, which, despite its ghostly name, is a vibrant ally for those needing pain relief. Harvesting this plant requires patience and precision, as it is often found in the shaded understory of forests, thriving in the dampness of decaying leaves. Its unique appearance, with translucent stems and delicate flowers, makes it a fascinating subject for herbalists and naturalists alike.

As you immerse yourself in wildcrafting, remember that each plant tells a story, a narrative woven into the fabric of its environment. By listening to these stories and respecting the delicate balance of nature, you become a forager and guardian of the wild places you explore. Every carefully harvested leaf and flower is a testament to your commitment to sustainability and reverence for the natural world. This journey through the untamed landscapes offers the bounty of herbs and a deeper connection to the earth and its timeless rhythms.

Herbal Vinegar and Oxymels: Ancient Remedies for Modern Times

In the quiet corners of medieval apothecaries, herbal vinegars were a staple, prized for their ability to preserve the essence of plants and deliver their healing properties in a potent form. Vinegar, infused with herbs, played a significant role in medicine, offering a means to harness the vitality of nature for health and wellness. Vinegar, infused with herbs, was used as a daily tonic remedy to maintain vigor and ward off ailments. Fast forward to today, and herbal vinegars remain popular for those seeking natural remedies. Their applications have evolved, yet their core purpose endures: to capture the benefits of herbs in a versatile and accessible medium.

Much like herbal vinegar, Oxymels boast a rich history, and many celebrate their effectiveness in supporting respiratory health.

These sweet and tangy preparations combine vinegar with honey, creating a soothing and palatable remedy. Traditionally, oxymels were used to ease coughs and colds, with the honey acting as a natural demulcent to coat the throat while the vinegar broke up congestion. In contemporary wellness practices, oxymels offer these benefits, providing a gentle yet effective way to support respiratory comfort. Their dual nature—both flavorful and medicinal—makes them an appealing choice for adults and children alike.

Creating herbal vinegar at home is straightforward, allowing you to tailor the blend to your personal preferences and health goals. One simple yet effective recipe involves infusing apple cider vinegar with rosemary, a herb known for its antioxidant and antimicrobial properties. First, fill a clean glass jar with fresh rosemary sprigs, then pour apple cider vinegar over the herbs until fully submerged.

After preparing the herbal vinegar mixture, you should tightly seal the jar, keep it air-tight, and store it in a superb location. Gently encourage the infusion process every few days. Once the vinegar has taken on the color and aroma of the rosemary, transfer the mixture to a clean bottle and store it.

Oxymels are equally easy to prepare and offer the additional sweetness of honey, which balances the sharpness of vinegar. Take a container with apple cider vinegar and honey to craft a thyme oxymel, then toss a generous amount of fresh thyme sprigs. The vinegar extracts the active compounds from the thyme, while the honey preserves these properties and adds a soothing quality. Shake the thyme oxymel often while allowing the mixture to steep for about 14 days. When ready, strain the thyme out and store your oxymel in a sealed bottle. You can use a spoonful to prepare respiratory support or add hot water for a comforting drink.

The health benefits of herbal vinegars and oxymels extend beyond their traditional uses. Herbal vinegar, which contains a high level of acetic acid, can help digestion. Acetic acid stimulates the production of gastric juices in your stomach, which aids in breaking down food more effectively. They also act as a natural detoxifier, helping to cleanse the body. Incorporating these vinegars into your diet can be as simple as using them in salad dressings. A drizzle over fresh greens enhances flavor and delivers the digestive benefits of the infused herbs, making every meal an opportunity for wellness.

Oxymels can become a staple in your daily routine with their immune-supporting properties. A small shot of oxymel taken each morning can boost the immune system, particularly during the colder months when respiratory issues are more prevalent. This practice not only supports health but also integrates a moment of self-care into your day, a reminder of the nurturing power of nature. As you explore the world of herbal vinegar and oxymels, these ancient remedies offer a bridge between tradition and modern wellness, inviting you to embrace their simplicity and effectiveness in your life.

INTEGRATING AROMATHERAPY: THE ROLE OF ESSENTIAL OILS

Imagine entering a room and being enveloped by a calming scent that instantly lifts your mood. This scent carries the subtle power of aromatherapy, which herbal medicine has intertwined with for centuries.

Essential oils, the concentrated essence of plants, play a pivotal role in this aromatic world, offering scent and therapeutic benefits. These oils work on two levels: they can influence our emotions and moods through the olfactory system and provide physical benefits when applied topically.

When you inhale essential oils, the scent may affect the limbic system in your brain, which is responsible for controlling emotions. This stimulation can cause the brain to release neurotransmitters—chemicals that help transmit signals in the brain—that can either lift your mood and make you feel happier or calm your mind and help you relax.

ESSENTIAL OILS PENETRATE THE SKIN, BENEFITING MUSCLES, JOINTS, AND OTHER TISSUES.

Among the vast number of essential oils available, some are especially notable because they are highly effective in many applications. We praise these crucial oils for their adaptability and the significant benefits they provide in various situations, making them stand out.

Lavender oil, for instance, is renowned for its calming properties. Some people often use its gentle, floral scent to promote relaxation and restful sleep. Whether diffused in the air or applied to the temples, lavender oil can soothe anxiety and stress, creating a peaceful atmosphere conducive to winding down after a hectic day. Eucalyptus oil, on the other hand, is a powerful ally for respiratory health. Its fresh, invigorating scent can clear nasal passages and ease breathing when diffused or added to a steam inhalation. These oils complement herbal remedies and enhance their effects, offering a holistic approach to well-being.

When using essential oils in your herbal practice, it's crucial to prioritize safety. Essential oils have a high concentration of active compounds, making them very potent. Because of this, applying them directly to your skin without diluting them first can cause skin irritation or other adverse reactions. To safely use essential oils, mix them with carrier oils (like almond, jojoba, or coconut.) When using essential oils, adults should dilute the oils. Add one teaspoon of carrier oil to two to three drops of essential oil.

Additionally, you should be cautious with phototoxic oils like bergamot and lemon, as they can cause skin sensitivity when exposed to sunlight.

Before using a new product, apply a small amount to a small area of your skin. Then, test to see if the skin is irritated. If there's no adverse reaction after a certain period (usually 24 hours), using the product more extensively on your skin should be safe.

Adding essential oils to your daily activities can be easy to do and pleasant. These oils require little effort and can enhance your experiences with their enjoyable scents and potential benefits.

For stress relief, consider creating a diffuser blend with lavender, bergamot, and ylang-ylang. These oils create a tranquil environment, perfect for unwinding after a long day.

For those prone to headaches, a roll-on blend can offer quick relief. Combine peppermint and lavender oils with a carrier oil in a roller bottle. Apply the mixture to your temples and pulse points when tension strikes, allowing the cooling sensation and calming scent to ease discomfort.

Integrating aromatherapy into herbal medicine enriches the sensory experience and amplifies the healing potential of natural remedies. By understanding the principles of essential oils and using them mindfully, you can enhance your practice and enjoy the myriad benefits they offer. As you explore the world of aromatherapy, remember that these oils are more than just fragrances—they are potent allies in your quest for health and balance. In the next chapter, we will explore the future of herbal medicine and how emerging trends and technologies are shaping this ancient practice for modern times.

By mastering advanced herbal practices, we deepen our connection to plants' healing power and refine how we integrate them into our lives. From synergistic blends to seasonal applications and fermentation techniques, these methods enhance herbal remedies' potency, sustainability, and effectiveness. The more we explore, the more we realize that herbalism is not just a practice—it is a lifelong journey of discovery, adaptation, and respect for nature's gifts.

As we conclude this chapter, we shift our focus toward the future of herbal medicine. While herbal traditions are deeply rooted in ancient wisdom, they evolve alongside modern science, technology, and global sustainability efforts. The final chapter will explore how innovation, research, and cultural revival shape the next generation of plant-based healing.

Herbal medicine stands at the intersection of tradition and innovation, blending centuries-old knowledge with modern scientific advancements. As more people turn to natural remedies, herbalism is transforming—embracing cutting-edge research, digital tools, and sustainable cultivation practices to meet the demands of a changing world.

In this final chapter, we will explore:

- 🌿 Scientific Breakthroughs – How modern research is validating and expanding herbal medicine.
- 🌍 Sustainability & Ethical Sourcing – The role of responsible harvesting and conservation.
- 📱 Technology & Herbalism – Apps, AI, and digital tools reshape herbal education.
- 🏥 Integrative Medicine – The growing collaboration between herbalists and conventional healthcare.
- 🤝 Community & Global Impact – The resurgence of herbal wisdom in modern wellness movements.

The future of herbal medicine is one of adaptation and growth, offering new opportunities to honor ancient wisdom while advancing the accessibility, efficacy, and sustainability of plant-based healing. Let's step forward into this exciting new era of herbal medicine and explore the endless possibilities ahead!🌿✨

The Future of Herbal Medicine

"Where ancient and modern herbal wisdom meets, discover a new frontier in wellness."

Ancient herbal wisdom meets the cutting edge of modern science.

Envisioning a place or moment where traditional herbal knowledge and practices intersect with the latest scientific advancements. It's a metaphorical crossroads where the time-honored wisdom of using herbs for healing and wellness comes together with modern scientific techniques and discoveries, creating new possibilities and innovations in herbal medicine. This blend of the old and the new can lead to a future where herbal remedies are more effective, widely understood, and integrated into contemporary healthcare.

It's a place where the past informs the future, and the possibilities are as vast as the fields of wild herbs stretching before you.

Ahead, we will delve into the latest advancements in herbal research. We will cover new and interesting findings, scientific breakthroughs, and innovations related to the study and use of herbs. The focus will be on how these developments are shaping the future of herbal medicine and enhancing our understanding of the healing properties of herbs. We will explore where scientific advancements validate traditional practices and expand the horizons of what herbal medicine can achieve—combining the old and new offers a glimpse into a future where the healing power of plants is more accessible and effective than ever.

Innovations in Herbal Research: Bridging Science and Tradition

Modern herbal research is a dynamic field where science tools lend credence to age-old practices. Genomic studies are unraveling the mysteries of plant DNA, revealing the genetic blueprints that underpin their therapeutic properties. By understanding these genetic codes, researchers can identify specific compounds responsible for healing effects, paving the way for more targeted and effective herbal remedies. This precision allows herbalists to tailor treatments to individual needs, enhancing the efficacy of traditional remedies.

Clinical trials are another cornerstone of contemporary herbal research. These studies rigorously test the safety and effectiveness of herbal treatments, offering empirical evidence that supports anecdotal claims. By adhering to stringent scientific standards, these trials bridge the gap between tradition and science, providing a solid foundation for integrating herbal remedies into mainstream healthcare. The validation of herbs like turmeric for inflammation or ginkgo biloba for cognitive support exemplifies this successful integration, reassuring practitioners and patients.

Interdisciplinary collaborations foster new insights into herbal medicine as herbalists and scientists collaborate in joint research initiatives. These partnerships enrich ethnobotany, the study of how cultures use plants, blending traditional practitioners' wisdom with scientists' analytical prowess. Conferences on integrative health practices serve as fertile grounds for exchanging ideas, where experts from diverse fields converge to share knowledge and explore new frontiers in herbal research. These collaborations are not just academic exercises; they translate into practical applications that enhance the quality and accessibility of herbal medicine.

New technologies are significantly changing the field of herbal research. These advancements allow researchers to understand better how herbs work, identify their beneficial compounds, and develop more effective herbal remedies. Technology is helping to modernize and improve how we study and use herbs for health and wellness.

Bioinformatics and advanced imaging techniques shed light on the intricate mechanisms of plant compounds. Researchers use bioinformatics to analyze complex data sets, revealing previously hidden patterns and correlations.

This approach allows researchers or practitioners to gain a more thorough and detailed comprehension of how specific processes or interactions work. It allows for a more insightful and in-depth exploration of herbs, leading to a better and more accurate understanding.

For example, in herbal research, advanced techniques like bioinformatics and imaging can reveal the complex interactions of plant compounds within the human body, providing more precise insights into their therapeutic effects and potential uses.

By leveraging techniques from biology, computer science, mathematics, and statistics, bioinformatics allows researchers to make sense of vast amounts of biological information, such as genetic sequences and protein structures. This interdisciplinary approach helps uncover patterns and insights that advance our knowledge of biology and improve medical research and healthcare. Advanced imaging techniques offer a visual map of plant compounds, illustrating their interactions at a molecular level. This clarity empowers researchers to refine and optimize herbal formulations, ensuring maximum efficacy and safety.

Despite these advancements, challenges remain in harmonizing traditional practices with modern science. Cultural sensitivity is paramount, as researchers must respect the knowledge and traditions of indigenous communities, ensuring that their contributions are recognized and protected. Standardization of herbal products is another hurdle, as the variability inherent in natural substances complicates efforts to create consistent and reliable formulations. Balancing herbal traditions' rich diversity with scientific methodology's rigor requires a nuanced approach that honors the past while embracing the future.

Reflection Section: Navigating the New Herbal Landscape

Consider how the latest advancements in herbal research might influence your approach to herbal medicine. What new scientific insights have intrigued you? How can you integrate these developments into your understanding of herbal remedies? Document your thoughts and observations in a journal, noting any changes you might consider in your approach to herbal medicine. This reflection will guide you in navigating the evolving landscape of herbal research, ensuring that you remain open to new possibilities while grounded in time-honored wisdom.

What is the importance and function of herbal medicine within the context of contemporary healthcare systems?

Herbal medicine is finding its way into the corridors of conventional healthcare, reshaping the landscape of treatment and care. Across the globe, hospitals are incorporating herbal clinics, offering patients an integrative approach to health that blends the best of both worlds. These clinics provide personalized care, where herbalists collaborate with doctors to create holistic treatment plans tailored to individual needs. Within these settings, herbal medicine complements traditional treatments, offering patients a wider array of therapeutic options. This integration enriches patient experiences and expands the scope of what modern healthcare can achieve.

TRAINING PROGRAMS FOR HEALTHCARE PROFESSIONALS ARE ANOTHER CRITICAL COMPONENT OF THIS SHIFT.

In the context of herbal medicine, this involves informing and training healthcare providers on the benefits and safe use of herbal remedies, ensuring they can make informed recommendations and provide holistic care addressing the whole person, including their physical, mental, emotional, and social needs, rather than focusing only on specific symptoms or illnesses.

Professionals trained in herbal practices can offer informed recommendations, ensuring patients receive safe and practical guidance when using herbal remedies. This knowledge bridges the gap between conventional and herbal medicine, creating a cohesive healthcare environment where patients benefit from the strengths of both systems.

The inclusion of herbal medicine in healthcare presents clear advantages. Herbal treatments are often cost-effective, providing affordable alternatives or supplements to pharmaceutical drugs. This affordability can alleviate financial strain on patients and healthcare systems, making holistic care accessible to a broader population. However, challenges persist. Regulatory frameworks for herbal products are often inconsistent, leading to variations in quality and efficacy. Safety concerns also arise, as the lack of standardization can result in products with unpredictable effects. Addressing these issues requires comprehensive regulations and rigorous quality control measures to ensure patient safety.

Case studies worldwide highlight the successful integration of herbal medicine in healthcare. Collaborative care models in community health centers exemplify how herbal and conventional treatments coexist.

By incorporating these herbal protocols, the centers aim to improve the patient's overall well-being and quality of life. This approach helps manage symptoms, supports healing, and provides a more holistic care method for those with chronic illnesses.

Integrative oncology programs (organized healthcare services and initiatives for patients with cancer) offer another compelling example. These programs provide holistic support by incorporating herbal therapies into cancer treatment plans. Patients report improved well-being and reduced side effects, illustrating the potential of herbal medicine to complement traditional cancer treatments.

Patient perceptions of herbal medicine are evolving as more individuals experience its benefits firsthand. Surveys regularly find that patients who use herbal remedies as part of their treatment plans are generally delighted with their results.

Many appreciate the personalized care and the sense of empowerment that comes with having more control over their health choices. By informing patients about herbal options' benefits and potential risks, healthcare providers can guide them in making informed decisions. This education fosters trust and encourages patients to explore herbal remedies confidently, knowing a knowledgeable healthcare team supports them.

In this dynamic healthcare environment, herbal medicine is no longer an alternative but integral to holistic patient care. As more healthcare systems embrace this integration, the potential for improving patient outcomes and expanding therapeutic options grows. The journey towards a future where herbal medicine is a standard component of healthcare is well underway, driven by a shared commitment to enhancing the well-being of all patients.

SUSTAINABLE HERBAL PRACTICES FOR FUTURE GENERATIONS

Imagine walking through a vibrant herbal garden, the air rich with the scent of diverse plants, each with its own story and healing potential. This garden represents a commitment to sustainability, a practice becoming increasingly vital in herbal medicine. Conservation of medicinal plant species is not just an environmental concern; it is essential for preserving the richness of our herbal heritage. As more people seek out natural remedies, such as herbs and other plants, the risk of collecting too many of these plants from the wild increases. Overharvesting can deplete plant populations, leading to a decline in the availability of these natural resources.

Ethical sourcing of herbs ensures that we respect natural ecosystems. By partnering with suppliers prioritizing sustainable harvesting, we can support practices that protect plant populations and promote biodiversity.

Innovative sustainable practices are emerging to address these challenges, offering new ways to nurture and preserve herbal resources. Agroforestry, a method that integrates trees and shrubs into agricultural landscapes, provides a sustainable solution for cultivating medicinal plants. By mimicking natural ecosystems, agroforestry supports biodiversity, improves soil health, and enhances carbon sequestration. This approach allows us to grow herbs alongside other crops, reducing the pressure on wild populations and creating resilient agricultural systems. Community-supported agriculture (CSA) for herbs is another promising model connecting consumers directly with local farmers. Participants invest in cultivating herbs and receive fresh, locally sourced products. This model strengthens local economies and promotes transparency and accountability in herb production.

Government incentives for organic farming encourage producers to adopt environmentally friendly practices, reduce reliance on synthetic fertilizers and pesticides, and help farmers transition to sustainable methods.

International agreements create guidelines and rules to help protect plant species and their natural habitats worldwide. These treaties aim to conserve biodiversity, ensure the sustainable use of natural resources, and promote international cooperation in protecting the environment.

These treaties guide national policies and encourage international cooperation by setting conservation and sustainable use targets. These efforts ensure that herbal resources remain available for future generations.

Examples of sustainable initiatives offer inspiration and practical models for others to follow. Botanical gardens focusing on medicinal plants are key to conservation and education. By cultivating rare and endangered species, these gardens serve as living libraries of herbal knowledge, preserving genetic diversity and offering research and public engagement opportunities. In addition to conservation, botanical gardens often engage in outreach programs, teaching visitors about the importance of sustainable practices and the value of medicinal plants. Fair-trade herbal cooperatives are another shining example of promoting ethical sourcing. These cooperatives directly link producers and consumers, fostering transparency and trust. By prioritizing fair-trade practices, we support farmers dedicated to sustainable production, ensuring their livelihoods are protected and their communities can thrive.

Resource List: Sustainable Herbal Practices

1. **Botanical Gardens Network**: Explore global efforts in medicinal plant conservation at botanical gardens worldwide.
2. **Fair-Trade Herbal Cooperatives**: Learn about organizations promoting ethical sourcing and fair compensation for farmers.
3. **Government Incentive Programs**: Investigate local and international policies supporting organic farming and sustainable practices.

These initiatives demonstrate that sustainable herbal practices are not just a possibility but a necessity. By embracing these approaches, we can ensure that our herbal traditions continue to flourish, offering healing and hope for future generations.

Technology and Herbalism: Apps and Tools for Modern Practitioners

In our digital era, technology is transforming all aspects of life, including herbal medicine. Imagine having a virtual herbalist at your fingertips or a digital library of plant knowledge that spans centuries. Online herbal databases have become invaluable resources, offering extensive information on herbs' properties, uses, and safety. These databases allow practitioners and enthusiasts to access reliable data that can guide their practice and deepen their understanding of herbal medicine—the therapeutic potential of herbs like echinacea or turmeric, supported by contemporary research and traditional wisdom.

The rise of virtual consultations with herbalists marks another significant shift. These consultations bridge geographical divides, connecting you with experts worldwide. Whether you're seeking personalized advice or confirmation on a particular herbal regimen, virtual consultations provide convenient access to professional guidance. This digital connection expands your support network about your health. However, as with all technology, ensuring that the herbalists you consult are credible and experienced is crucial, as the digital world can be a double-edged sword.

Software developers have created numerous apps and software to support herbal practice, each designed to make the world of herbs more accessible and user-friendly. Plant identification apps like PlantSnap use advanced image recognition to help identify plants quickly and accurately. These tools are perfect for seasoned herbalists and beginners, making plant identification less daunting and more precise. Recipe apps for herbal formulations offer curated collections of remedies, guiding you through creating tinctures, salves, and teas. With step-by-step instructions and ingredient lists, these apps simplify herbal preparation, allowing you to experiment and learn confidently.

While technology brings many advantages to herbalism, navigating its landscape thoughtfully is essential. The increased accessibility to herbal knowledge empowers more people to explore and use herbal remedies effectively. However, this accessibility also comes with risks. The internet is rife with misinformation, and not all sources are trustworthy. Unverified claims or inaccurate information can lead to ineffective or even harmful practices. It's crucial to cross-reference information from reputable sources and consult with knowledgeable practitioners when in doubt. Reliable apps and databases often cite their sources, providing transparency and accountability in the information they offer.

To integrate technology effectively into your herbal practice, consider using apps for personalized herbal tracking. These tools allow you to monitor your use of various herbs, noting their effects and any side effects. Maintaining a digital log lets you discern patterns and adjust to optimize your regimen. Online communities are another valuable resource, offering spaces for sharing experiences, insights, and support. Engaging with fellow herbal enthusiasts fosters community and provides opportunities to learn from others' experiences. However, always approach online advice critically and verify any new information against trusted sources.

Incorporating technology into herbalism offers a dynamic way to blend tradition with modernity, enhancing your practice and broadening your understanding. By leveraging digital tools thoughtfully, you can enrich your herbal experience, making the age-old wisdom of plant medicine accessible and relevant in today's fast-paced world.

COMMUNITY HERBALISM: BUILDING LOCAL NETWORKS AND SUPPORT

Imagine a vibrant community herb garden in the heart of a bustling city. This green oasis is a hub for learning, sharing, and growing. Community herb gardens are more than just plots of land; they are fertile grounds for collaboration and connection. Here, individuals pool their knowledge and resources, creating a shared space where novice and experienced herbalists can thrive. These gardens embody the spirit of community herbalism, where everyone has something to contribute and something to learn.

Local herbal workshops and classes further enrich the community, offering structured opportunities for education and engagement. These gatherings create a sense of belonging and foster a deeper understanding of herbal practices. Workshops focus on specific topics, such as tincture-making or plant identification, while classes could delve into the history and philosophy of herbal medicine. By participating in these events, you expand your herbal knowledge and connect with like-minded individuals who share your passion. This network of support and encouragement can be invaluable, providing guidance and inspiration as you explore the world of herbs.

Thriving community herbal projects serve as shining examples. Urban herbal cooperatives, for instance, bring together growers, herbalists, and consumers to create a sustainable supply chain that benefits all involved. These cooperatives often operate on a membership model; in exchange for their contributions, whether financial or through volunteer work, participants receive a share of the harvest. Herbal festivals and fairs are another testament to the power of community, celebrating the diversity and richness of herbal traditions. These events offer a platform for education, commerce, and cultural exchange, drawing in participants from near and far.

The benefits of community involvement in herbalism extend far beyond personal enrichment. Participating in local networks engages you in dynamic knowledge exchange and mentorship. Experienced herbalists share their wisdom with newcomers while fresh perspectives and ideas invigorate the community. Everyone benefits from the collective expertise. Additionally, collective purchasing of herbs and supplies can lead to significant cost savings, making herbal practices more accessible and affordable. By pooling resources, communities can access higher-quality products at lower prices, ensuring everyone has the tools they need to succeed.

Building and nurturing community networks requires intention and effort, but the rewards are worth it. Hosting neighborhood herbal study groups is a great way to start, bringing together individuals with a shared interest in herbal medicine. Collaborating with local businesses for herbal events is another effective strategy. By partnering with health food stores, cafes, or yoga studios, you can reach a broader audience and create opportunities for community engagement. These partnerships can lead to workshops, pop-up markets, or other events that promote herbal awareness and involvement.

Interactive Element: Herb Exchange Program

Consider organizing an herb exchange program within your community. Invite participants to bring herbs from their gardens, dried or fresh, to trade with others. An Exchange Program diversifies your herbal collection and encourages sharing and collaboration. This initiative fosters a spirit of generosity and cooperation, strengthening the bonds within your herbal community. As you participate, note the new herbs you acquire and how you incorporate them into your practices. This ongoing exchange enriches your herbal repertoire and deepens your connection to the community.

Embracing a Herbal Lifestyle: A Commitment to Nature and Wellness

Picture yourself waking up and smelling the soothing scent of lavender in your home. It's about experiencing a peaceful and calming atmosphere created by the natural essence of lavender, which helps you start your day with a sense of relaxation and harmony.

Living a herbal lifestyle is about making choices that align with natural principles. It means prioritizing natural remedies over synthetic ones for their health benefits and the deeper connection they forge with the earth. This lifestyle isn't just about what you consume; it's a mindset that values sustainability and simplicity. By choosing herbs for health, you reduce your reliance on industrialized medicine and embrace the wisdom of plants that our ancestors have used for millennia. Sustainable living practices naturally complement this approach. Whether growing your herbs, using eco-friendly products, or supporting local growers, each action contributes to a healthier planet. The herbal lifestyle is a harmonious balance between nurturing your health and caring for the world around you.

The holistic benefits of a herbal lifestyle extend beyond physical health. Natural remedies often enhance well-being, offering gentler, more sustainable pharmaceutical alternatives. Herbs like chamomile and valerian can soothe anxiety and promote restful sleep, while ginger and peppermint support digestion. The shift to herbal remedies often empowers you as you take control of your health with natural choices. Mentally and emotionally, tending to an herbal garden or preparing a homemade tincture provides a meditative escape from the stresses of modern life.

Furthermore, this lifestyle reduces your ecological footprint. By choosing local herbs and sustainable practices, you maximize your health decisions. An herbal lifestyle fosters a symbiotic relationship between you and the environment, where both thrive harmoniously.

Transitioning to a herbal lifestyle requires patience and openness. Start by gradually integrating herbs into your daily routines. Swap your morning coffee for a cup of invigorating herbal tea or add fresh herbs to your meals for flavor and health benefits. Slowly replace over-the-counter medications with trusted herbal alternatives under the guidance of a knowledgeable practitioner. Building a supportive herbal community can ease this transition. Connect with local herbalists, join online forums, or attend workshops to learn from others who share your passion. This network provides encouragement, resources, and shared experiences, ensuring you feel supported every step of the way. Embracing this lifestyle is a personal journey where small, consistent changes lead to profound transformations.

Inspiring stories abound of individuals who have embraced herbal lifestyles, experiencing healing and empowerment. Take Anna, who turned to herbs after struggling with chronic migraines. Using feverfew and magnesium-rich herbs, she found relief and reduced her reliance on medication. Her story is one of resilience and discovery, as she learned to trust nature's healing ability. Then there's Marcus, a community leader who advocates for urban herbal gardens. His efforts have transformed vacant lots into thriving green spaces, offering fresh herbs and a renewed sense of community pride. These narratives highlight the transformative power of herbal living, where personal growth and communal well-being intersect. By embracing a herbal lifestyle, you enhance your health and contribute to a more significant movement that values sustainability, connection, and natural wisdom.

Exploring Traditional Chinese Medicine: A Path to Herbal Mastery

Traditional Chinese Medicine (TCM) represents a rich tapestry of ancient practices and philosophies, offering profound insights into the healing potentials of herbs. Rooted in the belief that health is a state of harmony within the body and between the body and nature, TCM employs a holistic approach. It views the body as an interconnected system with intricately linked physical, emotional, and spiritual aspects. The concept of Qi is central to TCM, the vital energy that flows through the body, maintaining balance and vitality. When forces disrupt Qi, illness may occur. This belief underscores the importance of restoring balance through various modalities, including herbal remedies. Herbs in TCM are not merely used for symptom relief but are integral to achieving harmony and balance. They are often paired with practices like acupuncture and Tai Chi, creating a synergistic effect that enhances overall well-being.

With Traditional Chinese Medicine (TCM), practitioners use the principles of Yin and Yang to determine how they will use herbs. Yin and Yang represent the dual forces we must balance for optimal health. By understanding these principles, practitioners can select and prescribe herbs that will help restore balance in the body, addressing both deficiencies and excesses to achieve overall well-being.

Herbs are categorized based on their energetic properties—warming or cooling, drying or moistening—and their ability to balance these forces within the body. For instance, ginseng, known for its warming properties, is used to boost energy and vitality, especially in those with a deficiency of Yang. Conversely, chrysanthemum's cooling nature alleviates heat-related conditions, such as fever or inflammation. This nuanced understanding of herbs allows practitioners to tailor treatments to individual needs. The philosophy of Yin and Yang extends to the Five Elements theory, which links the body's organs to the natural elements of wood, fire, earth, metal, and water. Each component is associated with specific organs, emotions, and seasons, providing a comprehensive framework for diagnosis and treatment. This holistic approach empowers practitioners to create personalized treatment plans that consider each individual's unique constitution and lifestyle.

Herbal formulas in TCM are often complex, consisting of multiple herbs that work together to achieve a desired therapeutic effect. Practitioners precisely craft formulas, balancing the primary herbs with supporting herbs that enhance efficacy and mitigate side effects. For example, a formula designed to strengthen the immune system might include astragalus as the primary herb, supported by licorice root to harmonize and enhance absorption. This sophisticated approach reflects TCM's emphasis on customization and adaptability, ensuring that each treatment aligns with the patient's condition and constitution. While the complexity of TCM herbal formulas can be daunting, it is also a testament to the depth of knowledge and expertise that underpins this ancient practice.

Preserving herbs in TCM is also an art, requiring careful consideration of the best methods to extract their beneficial properties. Herbs may be prepared as decoctions, simmered for extended periods to extract active compounds, or as powders, tinctures, or pills for convenience and ease of use. The nature of the herbs and the desired therapeutic outcome guide the choice of preparation method. This attention to detail fully realizes the healing potential of each herb, offering maximum benefit to the patient. Mastery of these techniques is achieved through years of study and practice, reflecting the dedication and commitment required to excel in TCM.

By exploring TCM, this perspective invites you to consider how these ancient principles can enrich your understanding of herbal medicine. As you continue your journey through the world of herbs, let the wisdom of TCM guide you toward a path of balance and harmony where the power of nature is embraced and celebrated.

Exploring Traditional Chinese Medicine: A Path to Herbal Mastery

Throughout this book, we've explored the **power of herbal remedies** in restoring balance, strengthening immunity, and enhancing overall well-being. Yet, herbal medicine is as vast as the cultures that have practiced it for centuries. One of the most profound and time-honored herbal healing traditions is **Traditional Chinese Medicine (TCM)**.

For over **3,000 years**, TCM has utilized **herbs, acupuncture, Qi balancing, and food therapy** to promote long-lasting health. Unlike

Western herbalism, which often focuses on individual symptoms, **Chinese herbal medicine takes a holistic approach**—viewing the body as an interconnected system where balance is key to wellness.

One of the most fascinating aspects of TCM is its **deep understanding of Qi (life energy), Yin and Yang, and the Five Element Theory**—all of which influence our health in ways modern science is only beginning to grasp. Some of the world's most revered herbs, such as **ginseng for vitality, goji berries for longevity, and licorice root for harmonizing the body**, have their origins in TCM.

If you're intrigued by the ancient wisdom of Chinese herbal healing, the next book in this series will take you **deeper into the world of herbs, guiding you through its philosophy, essential herbs, and time-tested remedies.**

Ready to take your herbal knowledge to the next level? Discover **Stress-Free Living, and get your copy of** ***Stress-Free Living: Herbal Solutions for Wellness.***

Conclusion

"You are the ultimate authority on your health; nature's healing gifts are always available to guide and support you."

As we end our journey through the captivating world of herbal remedies, I reflect on this knowledge's profound impact on my life. When I first embarked on this path, a deep desire to empower individuals to reclaim their health through the wisdom of nature drove me. This book, "Nature's Healing Remedies: A Holistic Guide to Herbal Wellness & Vitality," represents the culmination of that vision—a bridge between ancient traditions and modern science, offering accessible and holistic approaches to wellness.

Throughout these pages, we've explored herbal medicine in depth, conducting a detailed and multifaceted examination covering various aspects. This exploration includes its origins and history, and how it is applied and used in modern times.

We laid the foundations, demystifying the basics of herbal preparations and safety. As we delved deeper, we discovered the remarkable properties of adaptogens, nervines, and digestive aids, learning how to harness their potential for resilience, calm, and vitality. We ventured into aromatherapy and topical treatments, uncovering essential oils and salves' gentle yet potent healing power.

Our journey also took us across cultures as we explored the diverse herbal traditions that have shaped our understanding of natural healing. From the ancient wisdom of Ayurveda and Traditional Chinese Medicine to the indigenous knowledge passed down through generations, we witnessed the universal human connection to plants as allies in health and well-being.

Embrace the process of experimentation.

As you reflect on the knowledge you've gained, I encourage you to embrace the emerging core lessons. First, trust your body's innate wisdom and nature's healing potential. Herbal remedies work harmoniously with your body's natural processes, supporting and strengthening its healing ability. By tuning into your unique needs and constitution, you can craft a personalized approach to wellness that honors your individuality.

Using herbal medicine does not bring immediate results or solutions. Instead, it involves a continuous process of learning and personal development. It emphasizes that understanding and effectively using herbs for health and wellness requires ongoing education, experimentation, and adaptation.

Embrace the process of experimentation and self-discovery, keeping a curious and open mind as you explore the vast world of plants. Seek opportunities to deepen your knowledge of herbs and healing.

Holistic lifestyle shift.

Finally, let this book be a catalyst for a holistic lifestyle shift.

Using herbal remedies is just one part of a broader approach to overall well-being. True well-being involves a holistic commitment to practices that support your mind, body, and spirit. This holistic commitment can include:

- Mindful Eating: Choosing nutritious foods and being present during meals.
- Regular Exercise: Staying active to maintain physical health.
- Stress-Reducing Rituals: Engaging in activities like mental mindfulness and meditation.

These commitments allow you to have a balanced and healthy lifestyle that nurtures every aspect of your being.

By cultivating a harmonious relationship with yourself and the world around you, you create a foundation for lasting health and vitality.

Reflecting on my journey, I am grateful for the countless individuals who have shared their wisdom and experiences with me. From the rolling hills of rural China to the vibrant markets of India, I have witnessed firsthand the transformative power of herbal medicine in the lives of people from all walks of life. I sincerely hope this book has ignited a spark within you—a passion for natural healing that will continue to grow and flourish.

So, my dear reader, I invite you to continue your herbal journey with curiosity, compassion, and wonder. Seek out new teachers, explore unfamiliar herbs, and trust in the process of self-discovery. Remember that you are the ultimate authority on your health, and nature's healing gifts are always available to guide and support you.

As you embark on the next chapter of your herbal journey, I encourage you to delve into the fascinating world of Chinese Herbal Medicine.

The ancient system provides vast information and distinctive viewpoints on health and healing. Traditional knowledge adds depth and value to what you have already learned from the book. The ancient practices and wisdom discussed can enhance and broaden your understanding of health and healing, offering additional insights that complement the modern information presented here.

By exploring the rich traditions of herbalism, you'll discover new ways to harness the power of plants for balance, vitality, and well-being.

I'm grateful for your time, attention, and companionship throughout this experience.

Your dedication to natural healing and willingness to embrace the wisdom of plants are testaments to your commitment to your health and desire to reconnect with the earth. Together, we can create a world where herbal medicine is celebrated, accessible, and integrated into the fabric of our daily lives.

May your path be filled with the beauty and bounty of nature, and may you always find healing, resilience, and joy in the gentle power of herbs.

With gratitude and green blessings,

Sage Meadows

🌿 Continue Your Herbal Journey: Discover the Secrets of Stress-Free Living

Congratulations on completing *Herbal Remedies: Unlocking Nature's Healing Power!* 🌿 By now, you have gained a **strong foundation** in herbal healing and how to incorporate nature's medicine into your daily life.

But this is only the beginning! 🌍 Across the world, Stress creeps into our lives in ways we often don't realize—disrupting sleep, clouding focus, and draining energy. But nature has always offered solutions. **Stress-Free Living: Herbal Solutions for Wellness**

Inside, you'll discover:

- **The science behind stress** and how herbs naturally promote relaxation.
- **Essential herbs for stress relief**, mental clarity, and emotional balance.

- **Step-by-step recipes** for teas, tinctures, and tonics to support daily wellness.
- **Ancient herbal wisdom, backed by modern studies**, for a holistic approach to health.

◈ **If you're ready to unlock the full potential of Stress Free Living, get your copy of** *Stress-Free Living: Herbal Solutions for Wellness* **today!**

Afterword

Reflecting on creating this book on herbs, I am filled with a deep sense of gratitude and accomplishment. This project has been a labor of love, born out of a passion for the natural world and a desire to share the ancient wisdom of herbal medicine with modern readers.

The path to completing this book was not without its challenges. From extensive research and meticulous documentation to capturing the beauty of each herb through photographs, every step required dedication and perseverance. I am incredibly thankful for the support and encouragement of my family, friends, and colleagues, who stood by me throughout this journey.

Herbs have been a source of healing and nourishment for countless generations. In our fast-paced world, it is easy to overlook nature's simple yet profound benefits. This book inspires you to explore the world of herbs, reconnect with nature, and embrace the time-tested practices of herbal medicine.

As we move forward, may we continue to cherish and respect the wisdom of our ancestors and strive to live in harmony with the natural world. I am excited about the new projects and look forward to sharing more knowledge and discoveries with you.

Thank you for joining me on this journey. Your interest and enthusiasm for herbs make all the hard work worthwhile.

Sage Meadows🌿✨

About the Author

Sage Meadows is a passionate herbalist, wellness educator, and advocate for natural healing. With a deep appreciation for Eastern and Western herbal traditions, Sage spent three transformative years living in rural China, immersing in traditional Chinese medicine's rich culture, customs, and ancient wisdom. Beyond China, Sage has also spent considerable time in Africa and various Asian nations, learning about diverse herbal practices and healing traditions. These experiences provided invaluable insights into the healing properties of herbs and the holistic approaches to wellness practiced across different cultures.

With years of hands-on experience exploring the world of herbal remedies, Sage seamlessly blends ancient botanical wisdom with modern wellness insights, empowering individuals to take charge of their health naturally. Through engaging and accessible writing, Sage simplifies the art of herbalism, making it practical and inspiring for both beginners and experienced enthusiasts alike.

Guided by the belief that nature holds the key to balance, vitality, and overall well-being, Sage is dedicated to helping others reconnect with the healing gifts of the earth. When not crafting herbal blends or leading wellness workshops, Sage enjoys foraging in wild meadows, cultivating an organic herb garden, and sharing knowledge with a thriving community of natural health seekers.

REFERENCES

1. Mount Sinai. (n.d.). *Herbal medicine information*. Mount Sinai - New York. https://www.mountsinai.org/health-library/treatment/herbal-medicine#:~:text=What%20is%20the%20history%20of,as%20early%20as%203%2C000%20BC

2. Huang, S., Wang, Q., & Wang, J. (2023). Current state of research on the clinical benefits of herbal medicine: A systematic review. *Frontiers in Pharmacology*. https://www.frontiersin.org/journals/pharmacology/articles/10.3389/fphar.2023.1234701/full

3. Johns Hopkins Medicine. (n.d.). *Herbal medicine*. https://www.hopkinsmedicine.org/health/wellness-and-prevention/herbal-medicine

4. Bloom Institute. (n.d.). *Common myths about herbal medicine*. https://bloominstitute.ca/common-myths-about-herbal-medicine/

The Gardening Cook. (n.d.). *Herb identification - How to identify herbs*. https://thegardeningcook.com/herb-identification/

5. Powell Gardens. (n.d.). *A guide to foraging with responsibility and sustainability in mind*. https://powellgardens.org/a-guide-to-foraging-with-responsibility-and-sustainability-in-mind

6. Chestnut School of Herbal Medicine. (n.d.). *Foraging for wild edibles and herbs: Sustainable and safe gathering practices.* https://chestnutherbs.com/foraging-for-wild-edibles-and-herbs-sustainable-and-safe-gathering-practices/

7. Urban Moonshine. (n.d.). *A wild foodie's guide to sustainable harvesting.* https://urbanmoonshine.com/blogs/blog/a-wild-foodie-s-guide-to-sustainable-harvesting

8. Grass Roots Remedies. (2021). *Infusions & decoctions.* https://grassrootsremedies.co.uk/wp-content/uploads/2021/06/Infusions-Decoctions-copy.pdf

9. Wild Spore Farm. (n.d.). *Alcohol vs. glycerin tinctures: Choosing the right solvent.* https://wildspore.farm/blogs/news/making-mushroom-tinctures2

10. Healthline. (n.d.). *A beginner's guide to making herbal salves and lotions.* https://www.healthline.com/health/diy-herbal-salves

11. The Herbal Academy. (n.d.). *How to make herb-infused oils.* https://theherbalacademy.com/blog/herb-infused-oils

12. Panossian, A., & Wikman, G. (2018). A preliminary review of studies on adaptogens: Comparison of their bioactivity in stress-related disorders. *Chinese Medicine*, 13(1). https://cmjournal.biomedcentral.com/articles/10.1186/s13020-018-0214-9

13. NIH Office of Dietary Supplements. (n.d.). *Ashwagandha: Is it helpful for stress, anxiety, or sleep?* https://ods.od.nih.gov/factsheets/Ashwagandha-HealthProfessional/

14. Bhattacharjee, S., & Ghosh, P. (2020). Antioxidant, antimicrobial and antiviral properties of herbal medicines. *Journal of Pharmacology & Pharmacotherapeutics*, 11(1), 45-52. https://pmc.ncbi.nlm.nih.gov/articles/PMC7767362/

15. Srivastava, J. K., Pandey, M., & Gupta, S. (2010). Chamomile: A herbal medicine of the past with bright future. *Molecular Medicine Reports*, 3(6), 895-901. https://pmc.ncbi.nlm.nih.gov/articles/PMC2995283/

16. Bodeker, G., & Kronenberg, F. (2012). Integration of herbal medicine into evidence-based clinical practice. *The National Academies Press.* https://www.ncbi.nlm.nih.gov/books/NBK92760/

17. Healthline. (n.d.). *9 home remedies backed by science.* https://www.healthline.com/health/home-remedies

18. Ginger Tonic Botanicals. (n.d.). *Creating an herbal apothecary at home.* https://www.gingertonicbotanicals.com/blog/creating-an-at-home-apothecary/

19. The Herbalist's Path. (n.d.). *Herbal first aid essentials.* https://www.theherbalistspath.com/blog/herbal-first-aid-essentials

20. Zandu Care. (n.d.). *Tridosha in Ayurveda: Balance of Vata, Pitta, and Kapha.* https://zanducare.com/blogs/exploring-ayurveda/understanding-tridosha-the-balance-of-vata-pitta-and-kapha-for-optimal-health

21. Better Health Channel. (n.d.). *Chinese herbal medicine.* https://www.betterhealth.vic.gov.au/health/conditionsandtreatments/chinese-herbal-medicine

22. National Institutes of Health. (n.d.). *Indigenous Native American healing traditions.* https://pmc.ncbi.nlm.nih.gov/articles/PMC2913884/

23. Heinrich, M., & Bremner, P. (2006). The European heritage of folk medicines and modern developments. *Phytotherapy Research*, 20(3), 163-171. https://pmc.ncbi.nlm.nih.gov/articles/PMC3638603/

24. Zhao, L., & Shen, Y. (2014). Synergy effects of herb extracts: Pharmacokinetics and pharmacodynamics. *Pharmacology & Therapeutics*, 15(2), 305-317. https://www.sciencedirect.com/science/article/abs/pii/S0367326X13002840

25. Gaia Herbs. (n.d.). *A guide to traditional herbalism across cultures.* https://www.gaiaherbs.com/blogs/seeds-of-knowledge/herbalism-folk-medicine

26. The Herbal Academy. (n.d.). *The craft of herbal fermentation course.* https://theherbalacademy.com/product/craft-herbal-fermentation-course/

27. Old Ways Herbal. (2019). *Ethical wildcrafting principles.* https://oldwaysherbal.com/2019/04/03/ethical-wildcrafting-principles/

28. Bharadwaj, R., & Gupta, V. (2023). Recent development of novel drug delivery of herbal drugs. *Research Progress in Pharmacological Sciences*, 2(4), rqad028. https://academic.oup.com/rpsppr/article/2/4/rqad028/7249912

29. Liebert, M. A. (2024). Sustainable health care: How traditional, complementary, and integrative medicine contributes to sustainability. *Journal of Integrative and Complementary Medicine.* https://www.liebertpub.com/doi/10.1089/jicm.2024.0754

30. National Institutes of Health. (2018). *NIH launches HerbList, a mobile app on herbal products.* https://www.nih.gov/news-events/news-releases/nih-launches-herblist-mobile-app-herbal-products

31. Weiss, J. (1982). Dermatology in the People's Republic of China. *Archives of Dermatology*, 118(7), 519-523. https://doi.org/10.1001/archderm.1982.01650140003001

32. Atlas Bar. (n.d.). *Unraveling the name: The origins and significance of monk fruit.* https://atlasbars.com/blogs/monk-fruit-explained/unraveling-the-name-the-origins-and-significance-of-monk-fruit

33. International Association for the Study of Pain. (n.d.). *Evaluation of the efficacy and safety of herbal medicine for treating work-related chronic low back pain.* https://www.iasp-pain.org/publications/pain-research-forum/papers-of-the-week/paper/121184-evaluation-efficacy-and-safety-herbal-medicine-treating-work-related-chronic-low-back/

34. Sotomayor, S. (n.d.). *The role of Ayurvedic diet and nutrition in achieving overall health.* https://aboutsoniasotomayor.com/5524-the-role-of-ayurvedic-diet-and-nutrition-in-achieving-overall-health-46/

35. TechBullion. (n.d.). *The science behind health supplements: What*

works and what doesn't. https://techbullion.com/the-science-behind-health-supplements-what-works-and-what-doesnt/

36. Wimbee Creek Farm. (n.d.). *Lemon balm.* https://wimbeecreekfarm.com/product/lemon-balm/

37. Med365. (n.d.). *Solal burnout 60 capsules.* https://med365.co.za/products/solal_burnout_adrenal_support_60_capsules

38. Maine Beans. (1985). *Maine beans.* https://core.ac.uk/download/230237070.pdf

39. Nao Medical. (n.d.). *Lemon and honey tea for sore throat: Natural remedies to soothe and heal.* https://aboutmanukahoney.com/lemon-and-honey-tea-for-sore-throat-natural-remedies-to-soothe-and-heal-nao-medical/

40. Frontiers in Pharmacology. (2023). *Harder, better, faster, stronger? Retrospective chart review of adverse events of interactions between adaptogens and antidepressant drugs.* https://www.frontiersin.org/journals/pharmacology/articles/10.3389/fphar.2023.1271776/full

41. U.S. Department of Veterans Affairs. (n.d.). *Adaptogens.* https://www.va.gov/WHOLEHEALTHLIBRARY/tools/adaptogens.asp

42. Healthline. (n.d.). *What are the benefits of Triphala?* https://www.healthline.com/nutrition/triphala

43. World Rainforests. (n.d.). *The Congo rainforest.* https://www.worldrainforests.com/congo/

Made in United States
Troutdale, OR
10/02/2026

55121918R00086